List of Contributors

Barbara Alving, MD, MACP
Professor of Medicine, Uniformed Services University, Bethesda, Maryland, USA

Mary Catherine Beach, MD, MPH
Associate Professor, Johns Hopkins University School of Medicine, Bloomberg School of Public Health, Johns Hopkins University, Baltimore, Maryland, USA

Howard Beckman, MD, FACP, FAACH
Clinical Professor of Medicine and Family Medicine, University of Rochester School of Medicine and Dentistry; Director, Innovative Strategies, Finger Lakes Health Systems Agency; Chief Medical Officer, Focused Medical Analytics, Rochester, New York, USA

D. Craig Brater, MD, MACP
Dean, Indiana University School of Medicine; Professor of Medicine, Division of Clinical Pharmacology, Department of Medicine, Indiana University School of Medicine, Indianapolis, Indiana, USA

Qiongzhu Chen, MB, MPH
Director of Dean's Office, SYSU Zhongshan School of Medicine, Guangzhou, Guangdong, China

Lisa A. Cooper, MD, MPH, FACP
James F. Fries Professor of Medicine, Director, Johns Hopkins Center to Eliminate Cardiovascular Disparities, Johns Hopkins University School of Medicine; Professor of Epidemiology, Health Policy and Management, and Health Behavior and Society, Johns Hopkins Bloomberg School of Public Health, Baltimore, Maryland, USA

Richard M. Frankel, PhD
Professor of Medicine and Geriatrics, Senior Scientist, Regenstrief Institute,

Inc. Indiana University School of Medicine; Associate Director, Center for Implementing Evidence Based Practice, Richard L. Roudebush Veteran's Administration Medical Center, Indianapolis, Indiana, USA

Shunichi Fukuhara, MD, DMSc, FACP
Deputy Dean, School of Public Health; Professor, Department of Healthcare Epidemiology, Kyoto University Faculty of Medicine, Kyoto, Japan

Guoquan Gao, MD, PhD
Professor and Chairman, Department of Biochemistry, SYSU Zhongshan School of Medicine, Guangzhou, Guangdong, China

Richard B. Gunderman, MD, PhD
Professor of Radiology, Pediatrics, Medical Education, Philosophy, Liberal Arts and Philanthropy, Indiana University, Indianapolis, Indiana, USA

Kaihua Guo, MD, PhD
Associate Professor and past Assistant Dean, Department of Human Anatomy, SYSU Zhongshan School of Medicine, Guangzhou, Guangdong, China

Paul Haidet, MD MPH
Director of Medical Education Research, Professor of Medicine, Humanities, and Public Health Sciences, The Pennsylvania State University College of Medicine, Hershey, Pennsylvania, USA

Judith A. Hall, PhD
University Distinguished Professor, Department of Psychology, Northeastern University, Boston, Massachusetts, USA

Thomas S. Inui, ScM, MD, MACP
Director of Research, IU Center for Global Health; Professor of Medicine, Indiana University School of Medicine; Senior Scientist, Regenstrief Institute, Inc., Indianapolis, Indiana, USA

Eric B. Larson, MD, MPH, MACP
Vice President for Research Group Health Cooperative; Executive Director, Group Health Research Institute; Clinical Professor of Medicine and Health Services, University of Washington, Seattle, Washington, USA

Enhancing the Professional Culture of Academic Health Science Centers

CREATING AND SUSTAINING RESEARCH COMMUNITIES

Edited by

THOMAS S. INUI

ScM, MD, MACP
Director of Research, IU Center for Global Health
Professor of Medicine, Indiana University School of Medicine
Senior Scientist, Regenstrief Institute, Inc.
Indianapolis, IN, USA

and

RICHARD M. FRANKEL

PhD
Professor of Medicine and Geriatrics
Senior Scientist, Regenstrief Institute Inc.
Indiana University School of Medicine
Associate Director, Center for Implementing Evidence Based Practice
Richard L. Roudebush Veteran's Administration Medical Center
Indianapolis, IN, USA

CULTURE, CONTEXT AND QUALITY IN HEALTH SCIENCES
RESEARCH, EDUCATION, LEADERSHIP AND PATIENT CARE

Series Editors

THOMAS S. INUI AND RICHARD M. FRANKEL

Radcliffe Publishing
London • New York

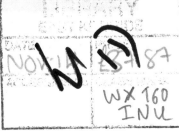

Radcliffe Publishing Ltd
33–41 Dallington Street
London
EC1V 0BB
United Kingdom

www.radcliffehealth.com

British Library Cataloguing in Publication Data

A catalogue record for this book is available from the British Library.

ISBN-13: 978 184619 523 5

The paper used for the text pages of this book is FSC® certified. FSC (The Forest Stewardship Council®) is an international network to promote responsible management of the world's forests.

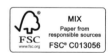

Typeset by Darkriver Design, Auckland, New Zealand
Printed and bound by TJI Digital, Padstow, Cornwall, UK

Contents

Contents

Mengfeng Li, MD, PhD
Vice President, Sun Yat-sen University (SYSU); Cheung Kong Professor and Dean, SYSU Zhongshan School of Medicine, Guangzhou, Guangdong, China

William L. Miller, MD, MA
Leonard Parker Pool Chair of Family Medicine, Lehigh Valley Health Network, Allentown, PA; Professor of Family Medicine, University of South Florida Morsani College of Medicine, Tampa, Florida, USA

David L. Mossbarger, MBA, MA
Senior Consultant, Public Consulting Group; Adjunct Professor, Indiana Tech; Lt. Colonel, U.S. Army (Ret.); Indianapolis, Indiana, USA

Bruce M. Psaty, MD, PhD
Co-director, Cardiovascular Health Research Unit; Professor, Medicine, Epidemiology and Health Services, University of Washington, Seattle; Investigator, Group Health Research Institute, Group Health Cooperative, Seattle, Washington, USA

The Relationship-Centered Care Research Network
Mary Catherine Beach, MD, MPH, Howard Beckman, MD, Lisa A. Cooper, MD, MPH, Judith A. Hall, PhD, Paul Haidet, MD, MPH, Thomas S. Inui, ScM, MD, William L. Miller, MD, MA, David L. Mossbarger, MA, Howard F. Stein, PhD

Debra Roter, DrPH, MPH
Professor, Department of Health, Behavior and Society, Johns Hopkins Bloomberg School of Public Health, Baltimore, Maryland, USA

Dana Gelb Safran, ScD
Senior Vice President, Performance Measurement & Improvement, Blue Cross Blue Shield of Massachusetts; Associate Professor of Medicine, Tufts University School of Medicine, Boston, Massachusetts, USA

Michelle P. Salyers, PhD
Associate Professor, Department of Psychology, Indiana University Purdue University Indianapolis; Co-Director, ACT Center of Indiana; Research Scientist, Regenstrief Institute, Inc., Indianapolis, Indiana, USA

List of Contributors

Anantha Shekhar, MD, PhD

Director, Indiana Clinical and Translational Sciences Institute; Raymond E. Houk Professor and Associate Dean for Translational Research, Indiana University School of Medicine, Indianapolis, Indiana, USA

David S. Siscovick, MD, MPH

Professor of Medicine and Epidemiology; Co-director, Cardiovascular Health Research Unit; Director, Cardiovascular Epidemiology Training Program, University of Washington, Seattle, Washington, USA

Howard F. Stein, PhD

Professor and Special Assistant to the Chair, Department of Family and Preventive Medicine, University of Oklahoma Health Sciences Center, Oklahoma City, Oklahoma, USA

Christine Tachibana, PhD

Scientific Editor, Group Health Research Institute, Seattle, Washington, USA

Hongmei Tan, MD, PhD

Associate Professor, Department of Pathophysiology, SYSU Zhongshan School of Medicine, Guangzhou, Guangdong, China

Edward H. Wagner, MD, MPH, MACP

Director Emeritus, MacColl Center for Health Care Innovation, Group Health Research Institute; Professor of Health Services, University of Washington, Seattle, Washington, USA

Michael Weiner, MD, MPH, FACP

Principal Investigator, Center of Excellence on Implementing Evidence-Based Practice, Department of Veterans Affairs, Veterans Health Administration, Health Services Research and Development Service HFP 04-148; Associate Professor of Medicine, Indiana University School of Medicine; Director, Center for Health Services Research, Regenstrief Institute, Inc.; Director, Indiana University Center for Health Services and Outcomes Research, Indianapolis, Indiana, USA

David S. Wilkes, MD

Executive Associate Dean for Research Affairs, August M. Watanabe Professor of Medical Research, Professor of Medicine, Microbiology and Immunology, Indiana University School of Medicine, Indianapolis, Indiana, USA

Linda S. Williams, MD
Research Coordinator, VA HSR&D Stroke QUERI; Investigator, VA HSR&D Center for Implementing Evidence-based Practice; Associate Professor, Neurology, Indiana University School of Medicine; Investigator, Regenstrief Institute, Inc., Indianapolis, Indiana, USA

Penelope R. Williamson, ScD, FAACH
Senior Consultant, Relationship Centered Health Care; Associate Professor of Medicine, Part Time, Johns Hopkins University School of Medicine, Baltimore, Maryland, USA

Minhao Wu, PhD
Associate Professor, Department of Immunology, SYSU Zhongshan School of Medicine, Guangzhou, Guangdong, China

Wenjun Xin, MD, PhD
Professor and Vice Chairman, Department of Physiology, SYSU Zhongshan School of Medicine, Guangzhou, Guangdong, China

Xia Yang, PhD
Professor, Department of Biochemistry, SYSU Zhongshan School of Medicine, Guangzhou, Guangdong, China

Yi Yang, MD, PhD
Associate Professor and past Secretary for Teaching, Department of Pharmacology, SYSU Zhongshan School of Medicine, Guangzhou, Guangdong, China

What's the Story?

A Composite Narrative of Success in Science in Academic Health Science Centers

Thomas S. Inui and Richard M. Frankel with Barbara Alving, Richard B. Gunderman, Shunichi Fukuhara, Eric B. Larson, Mengfeng Li, Bruce M. Psaty, Anantha Shekhar, David S. Siscovick, Edward H. Wagner, and Michael Weiner

THIS VOLUME IS DEDICATED TO EXPLORING THE RELATIONSHIP BETWEEN the culture and environments of academic health science centers (AHSCs) and their productivity in research. Other volumes in this series (*Culture, Context and Quality in Health Sciences Research, Education, Leadership and Patient Care*) have examined the environments of AHSCs and their excellence in education, clinical care, leadership, and responsiveness to policy. The authors of the chapters in this science-focused volume are drawn from a variety of North American AHSC settings, the National Institutes of Health (NIH), an academically affiliated research center in a health maintenance organization, an academically affiliated Veterans Affairs (VA) medical center, the school of medicine at Sun Yat-sen University in the People's Republic of China, the school of public health at Kyoto University in Japan, and a free-standing research network – a cross section of the heterogeneous organizational ecology of "academic health science centers." This diversity of locations, author roles, and national origin was intentional. The AHSC is becoming a "global phenomenon" not limited to any particular nation or region, or hemisphere. Though heretofore not present in these nations, AHSCs are emerging in Africa, England, and China.[1-3] The elements of the AHSC are situated in many different kinds of bricks-and-mortar institutions, and in some with no bricks or mortar at all.

By assembling this diversity of authorship, the editors of this volume (TSI and RMF) imagined that they could enrich the story that authors would tell about what enhanced the productivity of programs of science in AHSCs. Our approach to capturing this composite story was founded upon a theory of relationships and a method of inquiry. The theory of relationships posited, as others have done before us, that organizations like AHSCs are not properly understood as bricks and mortar, corporate entities, schools, or institutes but instead as *"people in a web of relationships who are engaging in 'conversations' with one another."*[4-7] This notion may at first sound rather fanciful, but consider the fact that your favorite institution was an idea before it became a plan with a budget and operating infrastructure (physical, social, political, or otherwise). Along its path of development, there literally were conversations about what should happen, would happen, and had happened. Even when the institution was a physical reality on the ground, it was populated by individuals who shared a mission, work collaborations, and a future. In this sense, the *most faithful* representation of an institution over time is as a web of humanity in relationship with one another, passing information ("in conversation") from one to another. If one can systematically tap into the narratives arising in such a web, the past, current, and future dynamics, values, and critical processes of the institution of the AHSC should be revealed.

The method of information-gathering we chose to explore AHSC science narratives for this chapter is *appreciative inquiry*.[8] Appreciative inquiry is founded upon the observation that the dynamics giving life to organizations are identified by hearing the *stories* of "work at its best." In such stories, people in organizations recount the specifics of situations in which they faced their usual challenges but persevered and found a way through, over or around these challenges, to succeed in their attempts to accomplish what had to be accomplished. The nature of these situations, the qualities of people in these narratives (the story teller and others), and the characteristics, policies and resources of the organizational environment are all significant determinants of success. The stories of these sentinel events, exemplars of what is working well in AHSCs, allow us to describe the work force, policies and situations that are responsible for AHSC success in the science enterprise generally.

The appreciative-inquiry interviews conducted for this chapter engaged one of the editors (TSI) and at least one author from each of the volume's components (foreword, introduction, chapters). The interview was a simple one. It was structured as follows:

- Please bring to mind an incident, situation, or circumstance in which you have felt at your best as a scientist (scientific program leader or in the science enterprise generally) – just like yourself, and highly successful. This situation could be yesterday or in the more distant past. It doesn't have to be a monumental event. The first situation that comes to your mind is the one I want you to recall.

- Now please tell me the story of that situation. [The interviewer listens and takes notes on the response.]
- When the story is told and any clarifications needed elicited, there are three probes.
  1. What did you bring to this situation that facilitated this success?
  2. What did the other people in this situation bring?
  3. What did the organization or its environment contribute to this success?

The interviews were 30–45 minutes in length, were digitally recorded, transcribed, and checked for accuracy. The contents of the interviews are summarized in Tables 1–4.

Examine each of these tables. *Reflect* on their content to appreciate the richness of the information. Table 1.1 suggests that the dynamics of success within AHSCs materialize in virtually every conceivable situation within these centers – in oversight of funded studies, mentoring interactions, writing grants, building trust and long-term relationships between research partners, convening and managing collaborative group work, recovering from an apparent failure or setback, making transitions in leadership of centers, seeking publication, translating information derived from research into practice, in laboratory dialogues, in efforts to improve clinical care, in relationships with patients and their families, and in conversations at posters at scientific meetings. The longer versions of these stories accompany each chapter in this book.

Table 1.2 suggests that the qualities of leadership in these situations are those of successful leaders everywhere. They include: courage, commitment, action orientation, perseverance, curiosity, passion, fastidiousness, generosity, saying the right thing at a critical moment, sharing gifts, envisioning possible futures for individuals or programs, having fun when "pushing the frontiers," sustaining research mindedness/valuing discovery, exercising curiosity, and setting aside hierarchical relationships to hear what others are saying. Some of these same qualities show up as critical characteristics of collaborators, protégés, bosses, friends, or others in Table 1.3. Success materializes in the interaction of leaders with others who are characterized as manifesting determination, good listening, honesty, open-mindedness, reciprocity, willingness to share resources, open-heartedness, risk-taking, different sensibilities, capacity to think about a future outside the present "box," and practical experience.

Finally, the policies and environments of AHSC that accommodate, facilitate, and support success in science are summarized in Table 1.4. Some of these environmental ingredients (e.g., financial resources and access to data) may be relatively unsurprising, while others such as strong institutional relationships with other organizations, policies of non-interference with principal investigators while imposing accountability for success, for example, would be unlikely to be found on a standard list of organizational policies and cultural attributes that relate to success in science. Other environmental factors that supported success included a culture of collaboration, pondering "big questions," codified policies promoting data-sharing, transparency, public-spiritedness, avidity for discoveries that improve care, and a democratic spirit.

The story that emerges from this inquiry about how science flourishes in AHSCs may be as simple as "recruit good people, get out of their way, and help everyone to feel accountable for success." Underneath this story, however, is a richer and more complex set of ingredients that account for success in the pursuit of any truly complex goal. As described by Westley, Zimmerman, and Patton,[9] they include: (1) Investing in relationships, especially those that span boundaries and organizational "silos." (2) Communication. Communication. Communication. (3) Emphasizing the core values and "vocational calling" that brought the people in a profession or organization (the "mesosystem") and to their work in teams (microsystems) in the first place – such as valuing health, and pursuit of knowledge and discovery of how phenomena in nature work. (4) Investing in the rising generation. (5) Creating a culture of transparency and integrity in the smallest work units and the larger organization.

The similarity of these deeper conclusions to the wisdom of others, such as Ernest Boyer, who have thought long and hard about "creating campus community" is unmistakable and worth reiterating.[10] Boyer, who was a distinguished and eminent American educator who served as Chancellor of the State University of New York, United States Commissioner of Education, and President of the Carnegie Foundation for the Advancement of Teaching, believed that university "enterprises" needed to come together in a coherent community of action for excellence in all domains to emerge. He suggested that university communities could and should be *purposeful* (sharing explicit and strategic processes), *open* (hosting diversity of all kinds, including of ideas and expertise), *just* (seeking to embody foundational values they share with society at its best), *disciplined* (hardworking, adhering to reasonable policies), *caring* (humane and supportive of human welfare), and *celebrative* (recognizing achievements, lifting up remarkable acts and careers). These *desiderata* for universities can be recognized in the stories of success in science that emerged from our chapter authors. At some level, these attributes may be widely recognized among leaders of universities within which AHSCs are nested. The recognition, however, of these foundational principles for organizational leadership, program management, and career advancement in the scientific enterprise of AHSCs seems new and fresh. The illumination of how these principles are embodied and come alive in the critical incidents that drive an AHSC science enterprise forward and inspire its workforce is a unique contribution of this volume.

TABLE 1.1 Appreciative Inquiry Reported Incident or Focus of Narrative of Success in Science

Brater: Mentoring a junior faculty member by illuminating possible future career avenues and the importance of finding a "niche" that isn't in a crowded career space.

Alving: Taking a deep dive into data to make an important decision about whether or not to stop the Women's Health Initiative estrogen trial in 2003–4. Working at the interface of science, government, and the public interest.

Shekhar: Confirming his hypothesis that hypocretin was operating as the "master neuroendocrine" transmitter in panic attacks by meeting and entering into a collaboration with two Swedish scientists who had collected cerebrospinal fluid samples for other reasons.

Larson: Helping a colleague overcome initial editorial rejection to move a "hot" finding into publication as well as into clinical policy and practice in the delivery system within which the finding arose.

Wagner: Convening a research team who loved to learn together. Science as a group process.

Li: Hosting a lab meeting in which the junior faculty could criticize and challenge me (the senior director of the research program and lab). It convinced me that I could do world-class research with this group.

Fukuhara: Recovering from an initial "failure" to introduce education for clinical research into graduate programs.

Gunderman: Being asked to give a eulogy at the funeral of a "stripped down version of a human being" (unfittest of the unfit, utterly devoid of what we think makes life worth living) who could easily have been forgotten or forsaken but was loved by his parents and community of others who took an interest.

Frankel: Building a trusting relationship with a colleague from a different discipline. We got to know one another by playing racketball, and he taught me the fundamentals of the game. From this beginning, we developed a highly functional research partnership and friendship.

Psaty: Using my best skills to write a grant that benefitted others by supporting infrastructure in the CHARGE [Cohorts for Heart and Aging Research in Genomic Epidemiology] network, not myself. This grant (from the NHLBI [National Heart, Lung, and Blood Institute]) got a perfect score.

Siscovick: Facilitating formation of research working groups in large, NHLBI-funded cohort studies that benefitted young investigators from multiple institutions by finding and building resources for mentorship.

Weiner: Using my expertise within a diverse team to respond to a clinical problem even though I was not "in charge" in a referrals and consultations study.

TABLE 1.2 Appreciative Inquiry Reflections on Contributions of Self to Success

Brater: Being willing to describe my own intellectual journey and the importance of intellectual curiosity (following your nose). Using "Have you thought about this or that?" probing and envisioning. "What is it that makes you feel excited?" Being able to listen at length without judging.

Alving: Courage of personal strong conviction in spite of split technical and scientific oversight in input on what to do. My commitment to the well-being of the participants. A neutral point of view on outcomes.

Shekhar: We had been working on this for 12 years, had done a series of animal experiments and had a good idea of what chemical might cause panic attacks, but no idea how to prove it. We were focused on about six chemicals. We (my lab group) were focused on the hypothalamus. When you stimulate this part of the hypothalamus, it is connected to all the parts of the nervous system and body – you get this sense of terror.

Larson: Promoting perseverance in dissemination efforts. I encouraged and supported reconsideration by the editors of an impact journal of the initial paper when it was rejected at first review. I said to the authors, "Don't give up."

Wagner: Thrust into a leadership role for a group of "intellectual powerhouses" all thinking together. I am a reasonably good facilitator of that kind of group science. We went out of our way to encourage "crazy ideas," push envelopes, not do the same old/same old, spread credit and rewards.

Li: Opening work groups to group ideation and disputation. I talked about my ideas, what I would like to do. I never tried to control this meeting, but everyone seemed really relaxed on this occasion. I tried to make the students feel as though they are the "masters of the lab."

Fukuhara: Realizing what's missing. My background in the Clinical Effectiveness Program at Harvard. I recognized that this kind of training should be part of medical education and training in Japan. It shifted my career from clinical medicine to research.

Gunderman: Curiosity. Always been curious about, been motivated by, big questions like, "What is the good?" "What makes us human?" "What are the limits of our capacity to love?" I am able to listen attentively. I will remember this occasion for a long time – I came away with an immense sense of gratitude.

Frankel: Willing to extend trust and share best gifts. I brought a microinteractional analysis background and a qualitative or "naturalist" approach. I was doing what I loved doing and developed a deep trust in my research partner. This was not a trivial matter since some of my doctoral research, my ideas, had been appropriated by a supervisor at another institution.

Psaty: Excellent writer and developer of group resources. I create research resources. I write well and know how to pitch things. I also have no need to be "in charge." I wrote the grant that provided support for infrastructure, including fellowship exchanges.

Siscovick: Stubborn (persistent) and able to think as a generalist. *Mazel* – be at the right place, at the right time, and say the right thing. In my own case, my passion and stubborn attention to my own topic of choice (omega 3 fatty acids, genetic risk factors, and risk of sudden cardiac arrest) led to seven R01s, grants that provided my support and support for four other young faculty investigators. In the context of large, NHLBI cohort studies, I worked to enable young investigators to form working groups within the studies, now a model adopted by NHLBI in other cohort studies. I take a generalist approach to cardiovascular epidemiology and prevention.

Weiner: Action-oriented and discovery-minded. I was trying to develop a new informatics tool that might improve the quality of care in the referral-consultation process, even though I was not in charge of the clinical domain or the information system. I was the research-minded person on the team who enjoyed problem-solving. I'm a bridge between domains of expertise. I'm also a do-er with an understanding of the constraints in the environment, and forward vision. I formulated a plan for action, but needed to be flexible. This project foreshadowed the RISP (research infrastructure grant focused on care improvement).

TABLE 1.3 Appreciative Inquiry Reflections on Contributions of Others to Success

Brater: Trusting mentees. They are confident that I will be honest and will focus on what's good for them instead of good for someone else or for myself.

Alving: My boss, the NIH Director Elias Zerhouni, "stood his ground" given input founded on evidence. He "had my back." He is also a very data-driven person. Good at listening. Straightforward and strong – he knew where he stood. All stakeholders (investigators, data safety boards, FDA [Food and Drug Administration], DHHS [Department of Health and Human Services], women participants needed to be informed). Strong trust between investigators and participants.

Shekhar: The Swedish scientists had been doing a project for years in which they were collecting cerebrospinal fluid samples from emergency room patients with various psychiatric conditions. They made it possible to test our hypothesis in real patients. They were immediately excited and even used their Swedish government grant to do the lab work.

Larson: Gold-standard mature methodologist. This was a non-clinician PI [principal investigator], so felt the need for support in a paper that focused on a finding in a clinical practice context. He was a scientist, so brought profound methodologic expertise and enthusiasm for discovery.

Wagner: Positive dynamics of group science. Everybody was contributing, everybody was learning, inventing new measures and new analytics, having fun. They relished being in a team and being immersed in team process.

Li: Willingness to express differences of opinion. The junior fellow challenged me, the PI. They had very good ideas – surprisingly good – and of high quality. Of the 30 members of the lab, only 5–6 embrace this approach. Everyone in the lab is smart, but these students feel responsible for the progress of the research in the lab. One day they will be the PIs and lead their own group.

Fukuhara: Honest assessment of problematic situation by a trusted colleague. Worked with an educator who confirmed that my approach was right, though the setting might not be.

Gunderman: An amazing family who refused to give up and give in even though their son could not speak for himself, or take care of any of his activities of daily living. The love his family showed for him was made all the more visible by the patient's fragile, brittle human life. The severely disabled adopted son was viewed by the family as a "child of god," here for a reason, and deserving of love.

Frankel: Long-term partnership with partner in research. He brought a clinical sensibility which complemented my skill set. He also manifested a clear commitment to communitarian values. I watched him in his practice be fully present in his work with patients. He loved his patients, and his patients loved him. He was a "straight-up" partner. It was 50/50. We later went to the mat for one another's promotions.

Psaty: Turn-taking from diverse expertise. Others have written very nice grants to support discovery activities in the network. The network brings together discovery and collaborative analysis of everybody's data for identifying genuine genomic associations. Others brought sample size and specific deep expertise in many sectors.

Siscovick: Access to intramural and extramural startup resources. Pilot funding from local foundations (e.g., Medic 1 Foundation and Clinical Nutritional Research Unit) and the Cardiovascular Health Research Unit, collaborative support from leadership from Medic 1, cardiology, and emergency medical services. They brought access to data, participation of the paramedics, and shared recognition of the importance of prevention.

Weiner: Practical knowledge of a clinical environment. The team of clinicians was aware that requests for consultations were getting lost and never fulfilled, but no one had a complete overview of the problematic situation. Other members of the team were practically-minded, collaborative, able to represent the needs and resources within their sectors, willing to be objective and fair-minded.

TABLE 1.4 Appreciative Inquiry Reflections on Contributions of Organization to Success

Brater: A culture of collaboration. The organization is highly collaborative. With a collaborative spirit, people want to help others. As Dean, my job description is to help others – full stop!

Alving: NIH well-situated in a matrix of interconnected key organizations. Good working relationships with counterparts at the FDA. We know our colleagues at DHHS and FDA. I could coordinate and arrange quickly the public communications and follow-up actions, such as those needed by the FDA.

Shekhar: I met my collaborators at a clinical pharmacology conference poster session in Paris. I used to try to "cover" hundreds of posters and meet dozens of people, but now I target just 6–8 posters and meet a few potential collaborators. The other "institution" is the CTSI – we are now in a dialogue with pharmaceutical manufacturers to find ways to block hypocretin – to treat panic attacks and/or prevent phobias.

Larson: Public-spirited, democratic organization with a founding commitment to research. There is an interface between organizational leadership and research center faculty that emphasizes mutual value. As one good thing happens, it begets another.

Wagner: A commitment to thinking out of the box and innovation. Program evaluation sponsor's advisory group was senior and conservative (e.g. in the context of the discussion of randomization), but the collaborative research group was committed to breaking new ground, developed its own culture of "creative juices."

Li: A non-hierarchical microsystem for science, even in a traditional institution. I tried to institutionalize this process in my lab. Everyone needs to feel themselves to be an equal. When I walk into the meeting, I tell myself, "Now I am one of them."

Fukuhara: Open space for innovation matched with accountability for success. Kyoto is a strong biological research institution, but it allowed us to pursue clinical research education. Kyoto leadership never interfered with our program.

Gunderman: Working in a context that allows him to ponder the big questions. Being around a family and community so committed to this young man.

Frankel: Open space for investigators to pursue their special interests. The institution supported faculty members to do what they wanted to do. Benign neglect and autonomy-supportive. "Do what you need to do to be successful."

Psaty: A culture of sharing key resources and transparency. Built-in principles and written policies about project leadership, data sharing, and authorship. Reflections on the need for transparency, opting in and opting out.

Siscovick: Inclusion of research in the mission of a public-service organization. Research is part of the ethos of the Medic 1 service in Seattle (emergency response system). We also have built mentorship and collaborative research opportunities into every project and network in which we are involved.

Weiner: Commitment to discovery as a part of improving quality of care. The hospital formed the clinical process improvement team into which a research and development effort could be usefully integrated. Within the hospital system there is a constant attention to quality of care and the need to serve the community well.

References

1. Mullan F, Frehywot S, Omaswa F, *et al*. Medical schools in sub-Saharan Africa. *Lancet*. 2011; **377**(9771): 1113–21.
2. Ovseiko PV, Davies SM, Buchan AM. Organizational models of emerging academic health science centers in England. *Acad Med*. 2010; **85**: 1282–9.
3. Shi Y, Rao Y. China's research culture. *Science*. 2010; **329**: 1128.
4. Stacey RD. *Strategic Management and Organisational Dynamics*. 3rd ed. Harlow, England: Financial Times Prentice Hall; 2000.
5. Suchman AL. How we think about organizations: a complexity perspective. In: Suchman AL, Sluyter DJ, Williamson PR, editors. *Leading Change in Healthcare*. London: Radcliffe Publishing; 2011. pp. 15–17.
6. Williamson PR, Baldwin D, Cottingham AH, *et al*. Transforming the professional culture of a medical school from the inside out. In: Suchman AL, Williamson PR, Sluyter D, editors. *Leading Change in Healthcare: transforming organizations using complexity, positive psychology and relationship-centered care*. London: Radcliffe Publishing; 2011.
7. Suchman AL, Williamson P, Litzelman DL, *et al*. Towards an informal curriculum that teaches professionalism: transforming the social environment of a medical school. *J Gen Int Med*. 2004; **19**: 501–4.
8. Cooperrider DL, Srivasta S. Appreciative inquiry in organizational life. *Res Organ Change Dev*. 1987; **1**: 129–69.
9. Westley F, Zimmerman B, Patton MQ. *Getting to Maybe: how the world is changed*. Toronto, Canada: Random House; 2007.
10. McDonald WM, editor. *Creating Campus Community: in search of Ernest Boyer's legacy*. San Francisco: Jossey-Bass; 2002. p. 3.

2

Challenges and Ingredients for Success in the Health Science Enterprise

A View from two Corner Offices

THIS CHAPTER COMBINES PERSPECTIVES ON THE ACADEMIC HEALTH science center research enterprise from two "corner offices." Craig Brater (Executive Dean) and David Wilkes (Executive Associate Dean for Research) describe challenges for research from the executive offices at Indiana University School of Medicine. Barbara Alving (former Director of NIH's National Center for Research Resources) comments on strategies for success from the perspective of an individual who provided leadership for the emergence of translation research from a "corner office" at the National Institutes of Health.

The Present Moment: Contemporary Challenges for Research in Academic Health Centers

D. Craig Brater and David S. Wilkes*

Craig Brater's Story of a Success in Science: Investing in the Future by Mentoring Young Faculty

When I was Chair of Medicine and also Division Head in Clinical Pharmacology, one of our young faculty who was in an oncology fellowship came to see me, asking whether I thought he should consider adding clinical pharmacology training to his preparation for a career. He liked oncology. He saw that he wanted to be in academics. The question as I saw it was, how do you build a successful career in a "busy space?" How can you carve out your own niche? I honestly can't remember now if he had some background in pharmaceutics, or why we may have been prospectively thinking about clinical pharmacology. It may have been just a generic discussion about career preparation, but we talked about how having a different perspective on oncology might give him some unique opportunities. Parenthetically, having a discussion like this might have been predicated on my own experience. I was on a trajectory to go into nephrology when during my training I met some of these clinical pharmacology types and thought, "Man, these people are really neat!" I liked the way they viewed the world and what they were doing. I then talked to some of my mentors in nephrology, and their advice to me was basically, in a nutshell, "You've got to find a niche that you can call your own and distinguish yourself. There is a boatload of nephrologists who are out there perfusing isolated nephrons. You could be in a large pool fighting to distinguish yourself among that group, or maybe you could go the clinical pharmacology path with a focus on the kidney and that would be totally unique." There was basically nobody in that space.

*   Department of Medicine, Indiana University School of Medicine

> This young faculty member enrolled in clinical pharmacology training, has been mentored along, has a big grant, and big recognition from one of the cancer organizations. I've seen him grow, mature and flourish to the extent he is likely to be a future leader here or elsewhere – hopefully the former! Seeing that kind of evolution with a little bit of hands-on advice from me from time to time, particularly when he was trying to figure out whether or not to do the clinical pharmacology part, has been terrific. When I look back at that from today I think well, gee, there are some people I really helped and maybe made a small contribution to their success. I feel proud and at least a little psychological ownership in what they've achieved to date but also the impact they will have in the future.

Research in academic health centers is threatened as never before. A surrogate measure of the challenge to an individual scientist is the age at which he or she attains a first R01 or equivalent. That age has crept up over the years and is now in the low 40s. This fact is complicated by a number of other variables such as the ever increasing competition to secure scarce federal funding for research, current weakened national and international economies that lead to uncertainty about future research budgets, dwindling philanthropic generosity due to economic woes, and declining state support for higher education. Furthermore, medical schools must rely increasingly on financial largesse from partner health systems at a time when their margins that have heretofore cross-subsidized research are shrinking. Collectively, the current state of affairs can only lead to overt pessimism about the future of research in academia. The paradox of this gloomy picture is that the opportunities for discovery, translation, and implementation have never been greater. It is indeed the best of times and worst of times. The current challenge to the academic health system is how to take these lemons and make as much lemonade as possible.

The stresses in the research environment mean most faculty members will have lapses in funding and institutions will need to make very difficult decisions about areas and individuals to support. More than ever scientists have a sword of Damocles hanging over them, and they know it. Similarly, leaders who have to make those decisions are under stress. On the one hand, everyone understands individuals need to be accountable but, on the other hand, they want to be supportive and encouraging. But being supportive takes resources and their lack is the root cause of the problems we are increasingly facing in research. Instead of dreaming about and executing growth, both individual scientists and people in leadership positions are faced with cutting losses. For both, such stresses can readily result in burn out, dropping out, being discouraged, and depression. People begin to question their own value. When that happens, the energy to write a grant application dissipates, the enthusiasm to inspire and mentor co-workers wanes, and a research program's virtual death spiral can become manifest.

Why would anyone pursue a research career in today's circumstances? Why would anyone pursue a leadership role in research? At the end of the day, research careers attract people because of the excitement of discovery. Even when we were in a more research-rich environment, individuals have always sacrificed to be research scientists. Some have hit the financial jackpot but the numbers are very few, so there has certainly never been a business case for this career path. The challenge then becomes creating and sustaining an environment where research is appreciated and celebrated despite the obstacles.

So how does one maintain a sense of what some might call pathological optimism about the future of research? That is what the culture of an institution is all about. The question devolves into what can be done at an institutional level to create a culture that is attractive to and supportive of the research environment. At our own institution we have tried to do so using a multi-faceted approach. Every other year we conduct what we call a vitality survey, the goal of which is to determine how our faculty members view their own world. This survey accomplishes several things. First, it tells faculty the School cares enough to ask. Second, it reveals areas that can be addressed to make their lives better. For example, one survey showed we were not adequately meeting mentoring needs. Acting on that need showed faculty the survey was more than a data-gathering exercise. We also seek faculty input in other ways including research strategies, areas of emphasis, expectations, and so on. Such an approach indicates the institution values ideas of individual research scientists as opposed to taking a purely top-down approach. When resources are available, groups of faculty are asked to participate in decisions as to allocation. All these efforts send a message that the institution values joint problem-solving. The assumption is even if news is bad, if individuals likely to be affected have meaningful input, they are better able to deal with challenges. Such an approach has led to many instances where the research enterprise has flourished.

There is no magical formula for how best to create an environment that will allow an institution to successfully navigate through the research challenges that face us today and in the future. It should be obvious that an activist approach and developing a culture conducive to research are essential elements. The chapters that follow will describe experiences and wisdom that will help in doing so.

Collaborations and Social Networking are Prerequisites for Successful Science

Barbara Alving

Barbara Alving's Story of a Success in Science: The Importance of Values-based Partnerships in Serving the Public Interest

I was the acting Director of the NHLBI from 2003 until the spring of 2005 and also the Director of the Women's Health Initiative (WHI). The estrogen plus progesterone hormone replacement arm of the trial was closed in 2002 by the NHLBI based on the unanimous recommendation of the Data Safety Monitoring Board (DSMB), but the estrogen-alone trial was allowed to continue. By 2004, it was evident to the DSMB and to us at NHLBI that certain of the stopping points were being approached in the estrogen-alone trial, although those end points had not yet been achieved. This is when great debates arose in the DSMB. The DSMB continued to debate what to do and finally came back to me, as the acting Director of NHLBI, with a split decision. Half said stop the trial and half said continue it. I told the NIH Director Elias Zerhouni about the data because any decision we made at NHLBI would have wide impact. Elias and I discussed this situation, and I expressed my strong opinion that the study should be ended. Elias decided to convene two extra, non-vested boards to review the data. After Elias considered the input of the DSMB and the two extra review panels, he also concluded that it should be stopped. When I reported this to the WHI investigators, they declined to be unblinded to the data, believing that the study should be continued, since it was never going to be repeated in any similar form in the future. They then began long conversations with Elias, who was thoroughly briefed on the matter and who stood his ground very firmly. We were thus able to bring the trial to a close with the ultimate cooperation of the WHI investigators. There were many stakeholders in this trial and in the communication of the results – the participants, the public, the specialty societies, the media, the scientific community, the FDA, DHHS, and the NIH. So this was high tension; however, we were able to get all of the agencies and organizations briefed and coordinated before the public release of the results. This was a very stressful time for me, but it was also an example of where we were able to pull together with the very strong leadership of the NIH Director. If the trial termination and subsequent communication of results had occurred in a chaotic fashion, it would have been an NIH-wide problem and detracted attention from all of the positive aspects of the estrogen-alone trial.

Subsequently, the WHI investigators re-consented the women participants for ongoing follow-up and research. The re-consent rate was very high, and numerous papers have continued to flow from the WHI, all of which will benefit women for generations to come.

Two fundamental characteristics of basic and clinical investigators are curiosity and the need for connectivity, as well as a strong sense of entrepreneurship, defined as the willingness to take risks in achieving goals. Translational investigators have a compelling need to go further: to see what is just beyond the horizon and then to bring it into view – to make it tangible and usable. Recognizing that scientific discovery has resulted in the ability to do complex science projects on almost any scale, they are now working in interdisciplinary teams to bring basic discovery forward into products and prevention strategies. In providing the environment for such collaborations, the National Institutes of Health, the largest public funder of biomedical research, as well as the academic health centers (AHCs), must navigate the economic, cultural, commercial, scientific, and political environments that are woven into the processes of bringing biomedical research to fruition.

Collaboration and Networking as Critical Factors in the Clinical and Translational Science Awards (CTSAs)

In the early 2000s, the NIH recognized, through discussions with leaders at AHCs, that efficient translation of the advances in basic research into clinically relevant outcomes required funding based on the demonstration of the plans for transformational change at AHCs. The CTSA initiative was developed amid anticipation and controversy, with the Congress as the ultimate funder giving tacit approval based on assessment of reactions of key constituents. The NIH weathered protests from basic scientists who were concerned that their funding would be entirely converted into a new large initiative, anticipated to be $500 million per year, as well as those who were the leaders of a more than 40-year-old program known as the General Clinical Research Center; these latter investigators feared the total disappearance of clinical research infrastructure, albeit a limited one, that they had known for decades. The CTSA initiative, the largest single initiative ever to be developed by the NIH, mandated that AHCs undergo transformational change to develop homes for clinical and translational research, as well as initiate degree-granting programs to teach investigators from diverse disciplines how to work together as interdisciplinary teams.[1] The academic homes provided the resources for translation, from biostatisticians to experts in regulatory affairs and technology transfer, to tools such as interactive websites for the development of Web-based protocols and information about investigators and core facilities at the universities.

The CTSA institutions also agreed to work as a consortium, sharing documents, course material, and knowledge freely with all AHCs throughout the country. The first CTSA awards were issued in 2006, and in an unprecedented action, the 12 CTSA institutions posted their successful applications on a website that was freely accessible to all.

With the growth of the CTSA initiative from 12 first funded in 2006 to a total of 60 funded by the end of 2011, came new ways to navigate within the consortium as well as new outlets for expression. A new society was born, known as the Society for Clinical and Translational Science with a new official Society journal named *Clinical and Translational Science*. In addition, the American Association for the Advancement of Science, wishing to capture the trend in the emphasis on translational sciences, also produced the journal *Science Translational Medicine: Integrating Science and Medicine*. The emphasis on translation and the development of the CTSA initiative has attracted attention throughout the world, with translational efforts beginning in countries such as India, China, and Australia, among others.

Ways to Facilitate Social Networking and Encourage Team Science

Junior investigators who have post-doctoral degrees can train in interdisciplinary teams at institutions with CTSAs; the investigators then receive master's degrees in clinical and translational science.[2-4] Pilot projects designed to bring interdisciplinary teams together are popular within the CTSA institutions, require relatively small amounts of dollars, and can lead to larger and more robustly funded research opportunities. NIH also recognizes multiple principal investigators on projects, and journals are now publishing the names of all of the authors of a journal article.

Social networking analysis tools are being developed and used in the CTSA institutions as well as in other institutions throughout the country; such tools can also determine links among investigators within an academic department[5] or in an institution or even across institutions.

The development of social networking tools and databases has greatly enabled team science; sophisticated systems are now available to search the Web and create connections among researchers based on variables such as primary and secondary research interests and geographical location, thus facilitating collaborations on complex projects that can move discoveries along a pipeline to the forefront of study. An example of such a system is VIVO, originating from Cornell University in Ithaca, New York, and designed to connect researchers with common interests across institutions throughout the nation.[6]

Social Networking in Laboratory and Community Research

Social networks and networking can be manifested in a variety of ways, depending on cultures, tools, and areas of need. Industry has led some excellent examples of social networking, which could also be called "crowdsourcing." For example, the Eli Lilly Company in Indianapolis has developed the "Open Innovation Drug Discovery" initiative in which investigators can submit to the company compounds of potential commercial value, thereby having access to phenotypic and target-based assays for diseases of interest to Lilly.[7] The investigator receives the data and then can develop further agreements with Lilly as appropriate. The Prize4Life non-profit organization,[8] dedicated to finding treatments and cures for individuals with amyotrophic lateral sclerosis (ALS), has partnered with InnoCentive,[9] a company specializing in open innovation, to find investigators interested in research on biomarkers, pathophysiology, and possible treatments; the organization awarded a prize to an investigator who has developed an assay that can serve as a biomarker for muscle response to drugs for ALS, thereby potentially enhancing the speed and efficiency of clinical trials for this disorder. Similar challenges have been successfully issued by Harvard investigators partnering with InnoCentive to award prizes to multidisciplinary teams to address type 1 diabetes.

Social networking in various forms extends throughout the fabric of society and is now being explored by biomedical researchers, in addition to social scientists. For example, a study of the Framingham cohort showed that the chance of becoming obese was linked with the individual's close ties with relatives, spouse, or friends who were obese.[10] This did not seem to be a neighborhood effect.

In a study in California attempting to find the cause of community clusters comprised of increased rates of diagnosis of autism in children, the authors found the diagnosis of autism in other children living in the neighborhood was due in large part to diffusion of information about the disorder in the community.[11] The power of social diffusion or networking can be used in multiple ways to disseminate and implement specific practices affecting health in the community.

Although the tools and technologies greatly enrich and enable social networking, one of the most powerful forms of networking at all stages of life and career development is the human face-to-face contact that occurs because of common interests or needs, which may already be known or discovered through the interaction. As investigators become more senior, social networking takes on the dimension of time and history of personal relationships. Senior leaders can then share their contacts with their mentees. Thus, acknowledging and building on the value of connectivity enriches and catalyzes progress.

AHCs are now being funded not only by the NIH, but by private investors and foundations, to collaborate and share their resources. The current emphasis on translation in the United States will take many forms and be funded in multiple ways. However, the NIH-funded CTSA initiative, regardless of its location within the structure of NIH, is likely to be the largest generator of new ideas in the use of social networking to accelerate the translation of discovery into the communities, both nationally and globally.

References

1. Zerhouni EA. Translational and clinical science: time for a new vision. *N Engl J Med*. 2005; **353**(15): 1621–3.
2. CTSA Consortium. Available at: www.ctsacentral.org
3. Rosenblum D, Alving B. The role of the clinical and translational science awards program in improving the quality and efficiency of clinical research. *Chest*. 2011; **140**(3): 764–7.
4. Meyers FJ, Pomeroy C. Creating the future biomedical research workforce. *Sci Transl Med*. 2011; **3**(102): 102fs5.
5. Merrill J, Hripcsak G. Using social network analysis within a department of biomedical informatics to induce a discussion of academic communities of practice. *J Am Med Inform Assoc*. 2008; **15**(6): 780–2.

6. Carey J. Faculty of 1000 and VIVO: invisible colleges and team science. *ISTL*. 2011; **65**(Spring).

7. PD² Lilly Phenotypic Drug Discovery. Available at: www.pd2.lilly.com

8. Prize4Life. Available at: www.prize4life.org

9. InnoCentive. Available at: www.innocentive.com

10. Christakis NA, Fowler JH. The spread of obesity in a large social network over 32 years. *N Engl J Med*. 2007; **357**(4): 370–9.

11. Liu KY, King M, Bearman PS. Social influence and the autism epidemic. *AJS*. 2010; **115**(5): 1387–434.

3

Breaking out of the Silos in the Heartland

Making a Clinical and Translational Science Award Program Sing in Indiana

*Anantha Shekhar**

Anantha Shekhar's Story of a Success in Science: Serendipity to the Rescue

My colleagues and I had done a whole series of animal experiments trying to identify what chemical might cause panic attacks. We knew exactly which part of the brain activates in panic attacks; we also knew in experiments what some of the signatures of those cells were, and had a top-candidate neuropeptide in mind – hypocretin. Hypocretin is involved in lots of diurnal rhythms and regulates our sleep/wake cycles, appetite, and our energy. It's an arousal chemical. It goes up when we wake up and goes down when we go to sleep.

This was a good hypothesis, but we had no way to confirm it. As it happened, I attended a poster session at a clinical pharmacology meeting in Paris. One poster that attracted me was being presented by a senior professor and a junior colleague from Sweden who had data on serotonin and some

* Indiana Clinical and Translational Sciences Institute
  Indiana University School of Medicine
  Indianapolis, Indiana 46202

other neurotransmitter levels in the cerebrospinal fluid (CSF) of people with chronic alcohol abuse. I was simply interested in looking at the data they were presenting. As we started talking, I realized they had collected and saved hundreds of CSF samples on emergency room patients over eight years, including people with panic attacks. They had published a few papers looking at a variety of chemicals in small numbers of patients. When I asked if they had studied panic attacks they said, "Oh yes! – we have CSF from hundreds of patients with all kinds of psychiatric conditions." It was a totally serendipitous matching of interests. We ended up collaborating with this group and did a condition-blinded assay of different chemicals that are high or low in CSF in cohorts of substance abuse and other non-psychiatric diagnoses, patients with depression and suicidal behavior, and finally patients with acute panic attacks. It turned out that it was only the panic group and none of the others who had two to three-fold increases in their CSF of our candidate chemical hypocretin. It was like the gods had spoken and said, "Your guess was right!" We were able to publish this finding in *Nature*.

We build too many walls and not enough bridges.

— Sir Isaac Newton

At the basic end of the biomedical research spectrum, we are in the midst of enormous gains that are fundamentally transforming our understanding of human biology, with sequencing of the genome, discovery of scores of novel biochemical pathways and improved ability to elucidate the potential molecular mechanisms underlying complex human diseases. Yet, our successes at generating actual clinical interventions from these basic science gains have been steadily declining. Any major discovery at the basic level takes 10 years or more before it can become an approved drug, and then it takes an additional decade or more before such an approved therapy is integrated into routine practice.[1,2] The industries that bring new discoveries into the market place as new therapies, devices, or diagnostic tests are in the midst of a crisis, with exponentially increasing costs, regulatory barriers, and long development time burdens. Furthermore, the impact of some of the innovations that do reach the market are plagued by the enormous delays in their implementation into routine disease management, due in part to limited health services and health outcomes research. From the foregoing, it was evident that biomedical research needed a paradigm shift in order to move forward. The key goal for the new paradigm was to devise methodologies that would facilitate the "translation" of research findings into practical clinical interventions.

Defining Translational Biomedical Science

An essential first step was to inventory and bring together the disparate, some-what loosely defined and variously successful methodologies that were being used at the intersection of bench, clinical, and population research arenas into a single "academic home" with specific resources to make sure that the best talents would be attracted to work together in this "new" field of research. These "homes" needed to be established at the leading academic health centers that could foster the interaction among scientists working at every level of the biomedical research spectrum. They would be designed to accelerate emerging basic research find-ings into new therapies and then to ensure their rapid adoption into practice. This new mechanism needed to bring together existing best practices and also discover new ways of rapidly transporting new molecules, devices, technologies, or evidence-based interventions into testing, validating, and adoption into human health-care practices. It needed to bring back the evidence that arises from clinical trials and outcomes research to create new questions and approaches to be addressed by basic science researchers. In essence, what was needed to foster such a new paradigm was the creation of a newly aligned field of science, "Translational Biomedical Science."

Translational Science, thus conceived, would develop fields of study that focus on solving the "translational" challenges; that is, identifying the chasms that exist among basic scientists of different backgrounds, clinicians (physicians, nurses, dentists, and veterinarians), allied health professionals (pharmacists, therapists, technologists), biomedical engineers, behavioral and social scientists, epidemi-ologists, and ultimately consumers, and build bridges to help transcend those barriers. This type of thinking eventually resulted in a major initiative from the National Institutes of Health in 2006, called Clinical and Translational Science Awards (CTSA) to establish regional "homes" for innovative translational research in 60 academic medical centers (AMCs) across the United States.[3]

Challenges of Translational Biomedical Sciences

When one looked at delays in the translation of research findings into new therapies or routinely implemented interventions, three major barriers seem to be critical: lack of a trained research workforce knowledgeable about translational processes; barriers caused by complex regulatory requirements with poorly coordinated infrastructure; and barriers resulting from organizational silos within institutions.[4] For example, studies showed that when attempting to begin multicenter, clinical trials for answering an efficacy or best practice question, less than a quarter of the sites were able to get local Institutional Ethics Review Board (IRB) approvals, and only 52% completed the contract agreements within 6 months.[5] Most clinical studies in AMCs have difficulty enrolling patients and fully half or more studies never meet their full enrollment goals. This was one of the key challenges that needed to be addressed by the national CTSA network.[6,7]

Translational Sciences: The Indiana Vision

The timing of the CTSA announcement was ideal for the Indiana University School of Medicine. In 2000, IUSM was awarded a $155 million grant from the Lilly Endowment to establish the Indiana Genomics Initiative (INGEN). This was the largest single grant ever received by Indiana University and awarded by the Lilly Endowment. INGEN represented a cooperative effort of scientists at IU, Purdue University (PU), and the University of Notre Dame, and was devoted to establishing research resources and training related to the Human Genome Project. It consisted of six thematic programs (genomics, bioinformatics, bioethics, education, training, and medical informatics) and several technology cores (information technology, genotyping and gene expression, proteomics, cell and protein expression, in vivo imaging, human expression, animal modeling, and technology transfer). The advanced information technology facilities for INGEN consisted of five components: supercomputing, massive data storage, advanced visualization, high-speed networking, and staff support. Once initiated, IU's facilities, resources, and expertise had began to gain national and international recognition.

In late 2006, I was tasked by the Dean of IUSM, Craig Brater, to lead our effort to secure a CTSA award. Based on the successful INGEN initiative, it was immediately evident to me that the most logical approach would be to bring together the resources available within Indiana and Purdue Universities, link them with critical non-academic stakeholders across the state and present our organization as a statewide translational laboratory to the NIH CTSA network. Equally important to the local stakeholders, this would create a vibrant Indiana Clinical and Translational Science Institute (CTSI) in Indiana, which could become the regional engine for "Translational Sciences" research and training.

In order to "sell" this vision of a statewide "laboratory" to both academic schools, and the wide range of stakeholders such as Clarian Health Partners (the state's largest hospital network and health-care provider, recently renamed IU Health), Lilly (a top 10 big Pharma), Cook Industries (a top 10 device manufacturer) and WellPoint (the nation's largest private health insurance company), our concept of Translational Sciences needed to paint the broadest possible canvas.

It should be envisioned as supporting the smooth flow of ideas and collaborations along an iterative cycle of Translation (T) valleys, starting with studies that take "bench" findings to controlled clinical trials at the "bedside" (T1); moving to studies that test results obtained in controlled clinical settings into larger communities (T2); leading to studies that translate into practice and clinical effectiveness (T3); and finally bringing the knowledge gained from population responses back to the "laboratory" for further study and refinement (T4), thus beginning the transformation cycle again. We called this our translational cycle[8] (*see* Figure 3.1).

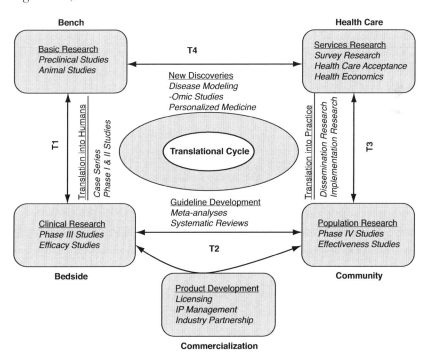

FIGURE 3.1 Schematic diagram of the Translational Circle as conceived for the Indiana CTSI

The Hard Work of Building
••••••••••••••••••••••••••••••

With such a broad canvas in mind, beginning in early January 2007, I began to meet individually with key stakeholders across the state. These included: leading researchers, directors of many academic divisions and institutes, administrators of the major teaching hospitals, biomedical industry leaders, community partner groups, state health officials, philanthropic foundations, and members of local economic development groups. I participated in more than 250 individual and small group meetings over a 6-month period to garner important individual guidance and buy-in from a broad range of Indiana communities for designing and developing the CTSI. By February of 2007, I had recruited a "core working group" of academic and non-academic biomedical leaders, who began tackling the task of designing a comprehensive Indiana CTSI in biweekly 3-hour meetings with specific sub-group work assignments between meetings. The work group, which began with membership of about 25 individuals, had increased to its final size of 56 members by April 2007. Each of the members was eager to participate and, in a number of cases, voluntarily requested membership. This unprecedented level of active participation by members of diverse schools from IU, PU, and non-academic communities, during 21 such weekly to biweekly meetings held from January 30 to July 24, 2007, provided the material from which the design of the Indiana CTSI emerged.

Based on our "translational cycle" (Figure 3.1), we developed unique programs within the Indiana CTSI to address each of these "inflection" steps within the cycle. The Indiana CTSI was designed to be the driving force for translational science at all the partner institutions, including the IU Health Sciences schools located at Indiana University Purdue University Indianapolis (IUPUI), Purdue University, and IU-Bloomington, and many community partners throughout Indiana. We were out of our silos!

Once we defined the broad goals and structure of the Indiana CTSI, we formed an executive leadership group to represent the broad subdivisions of this structure. In consultations with the executive group and each university's leadership, specific choices of the individual programs were made. These program leaders formed core program writing teams which were comprised of leaders in their respective fields. Multiple drafts were prepared and reviewed by assigned members of the entire work group. In addition, we solicited external input from three consultants who were senior leaders of already funded Clinical and Translational Sciences Institutes at other academic institutions across the country. These CTSA leaders visited Indiana on two occasions, interacted with the

CTSI work groups and university leadership, and provided us with independent assessments and advice on our strategy to build the Indiana CTSI. This methodical and arduous process, involving scores of faculty and thousands of volunteered hours of expert time, along with an investment of over $300 000 to support the planning process by IUSM, created a truly transformational Institute of Clinical and Translational Sciences for Indiana. Eventually, the University of Notre Dame also joined this academic consortium in 2008.

What Unique Assets make a Statewide Translational Laboratory?

The Indiana CTSI was designed with an ambitious agenda, the ability to shape an entire state's biomedical translational efforts, and access to most of the state's population health data through medical informatics capabilities. It would be capable of innovation and influence in shaping public and private health services of the whole state through partnerships with the Governor's office, state legislature, state service agencies and health insurance programs. In short, the Indiana CTSI model provided to the national network of CTSAs a true statewide laboratory to experiment with innovative methods aimed at transforming research in health economics, health-care delivery, and health policy. To this end, it brought together many unique and innovative assets, as follows.

1. Nationally and internationally recognized health informatics strengths of the Regenstrief Institute: the Indiana CTSI is home to world leaders in medical informatics and health services research, and is connected to the Indiana Health Information Exchange[9] (IHIE; Chang et al., 2010) and one of the nation's leading practice-based research networks (PBRNs; Kho et al., 2007).[10]

2. Unusual willingness to collaborate by all major private and public hospital systems in the region. This includes Indiana University Health, the university affiliated private health provider that is ranked as one of the largest health provider systems in the country, and Wishard Memorial Hospital and its parent organization Health Hospital Corporation form one of the two largest publicly owned community health systems in the country.

3. Indiana's statewide life science movement led by local universities and businesses. Indiana is home to a life sciences industry with annual expenditures estimated to be approximately $26 billion.[11] Life sciences jobs represent 9% of all employment and 20% of the tax base. In 2002, Central Indiana corporate

leaders, the city of Indianapolis, Indiana University, Purdue University, Eli Lilly and Co. and the Indiana Health Industry Forum created the Central Indiana Life Sciences Initiative, BioCrossroads. It is Indiana's initiative to help grow the life sciences economy in Indiana. BioCrossroads provides commercial investment and grant funding to emerging life science initiatives, launches new life sciences businesses, forms and expands collaborations and partnerships among Indiana's life science institutions, expands science education and workforce development, and markets Indiana's life sciences industry.

4. Population diversity with large urban, rural, and ethnic subpopulations. A truly extraordinary community medical record system in IHIE that brings together personal health information from more than 6 million people, providing a translational research database that is unparalleled anywhere else in the country. The Indiana population is not only diverse, but, unfortunately, it is also rich in conditions of interest (obesity, diabetes, heart disease, and others).

5. Through its partnership with Purdue, the Indiana CTSI also brought nationally and internationally recognized programs in veterinary medicine, nanomedicine, and biomedical engineering to the national CTSA network.

6. A unique statewide network (I-light) managed by Indiana University that provides high-speed network capability for in-state communications among participating sites, as well as advanced cyber infrastructure to support massive data analysis and simulations required to enable transformative breakthroughs in clinical research.

Design of the Indiana CTSI

The overarching goal of the Indiana CTSI was to create an environment that facilitates clinical and translational science research. Its mission is: "To increase translational biomedical research and improve the health of the people of Indiana and beyond." To this end, we focused on and developed new mechanisms to accelerate translational research; enhanced educational programs to train translational researchers; designed a community engagement activity, the Community Health Enhancement Program (CHEP) to produce effective and bidirectional community partnerships; and streamlined all available research infrastructure to accelerate translational projects. The critical link through all of this was a new communication platform called the CTSI HUB program, enabling all parties to interact in a facile manner. In summary, the Indiana CTSI bridged together the resources of academic, commercial, and community groups across the state. It provided a "home" to investigators with expertise in a wide range of fields relevant to clinical and translational research.

Building an "ideal" home for clinical and translational research activities presents significant challenges but also provides extraordinary opportunities to rethink one's institutional research enterprise. As noted above, we proceeded to systematically rethink and reorganize our entire research enterprise. We began with input from the research community within and outside the academic institutions of Indiana. Information was distilled through a series of weekly workshops with a core group of research leaders from Indiana and Purdue Universities, as well as various representatives of local corporations, not-for-profit organizations, and other interest groups. It resulted in defining the goals for the Indiana CTSI. Figure 3.2 provides an overview of the entire CTSI, its participant institutions, and its five specific goals along with the individual programs designed to achieve the stated goals.

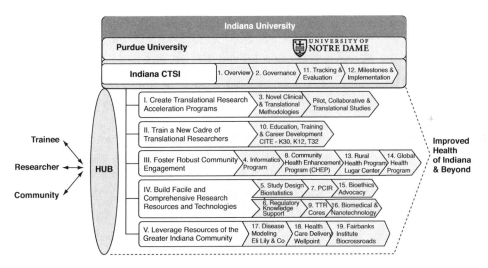

FIGURE 3.2 The five goals of the Indiana CTSI

The five goals of the Indiana CTSI are to:

I. Create Translational Research Acceleration Programs and Support Pilot Projects by providing investigators and consumers with strategic leadership and mentorship to identify, evaluate, and support innovative and important pilot research at each step of the translational cycle.

II. Train a new cadre of Translational Researchers by strengthening existing programs and creating new ones to educate trainees and engage faculty in the translational sciences.

III. Foster Robust Community Engagement by creating novel programs with bidirectional participation (i.e., from academia to the community and back again), such as the Indiana Community Health Enhancement Program and pilot programs in Rural and Global Health.

IV. Build Facile and Comprehensive Research Resources and Technologies by transforming the existing and new research infrastructure into innovative programs such as the Participant and Clinical Interaction Resources (PCIR), Translational Technology Resources (TTR), Research Ethics, Biostatistics and Design Program (BDP), and others to facilitate the translation of research.

V. Leverage the Resources of the Greater Indiana Community by connecting to a broad array of resources from multiple partner institutions throughout the state of Indiana, such as the novel modeling and clinical pharmacology training program with Eli Lilly; Health Economics Program with WellPoint; Global Health Program with our long-established collaboration with Moi Medical School in Kenya; and the Indiana Longitudinal Health Research Project for condition-targeted collections of human biologic materials within the Fairbanks Institute, a local non-profit organization.

Crisis at Birth: Fairbanks Foundation to the Rescue!

Our CTSA application was reviewed in early 2008. The NIH panel was very enthusiastic about our plans and the likelihood of our success in enhancing translational research in Indiana. However, due to federal budget limitations, the NIH was only able to fund about half of the total costs. This meant that we were starting off with nearly $20 million (or 35% reduction in the total five-year budget) less than we had anticipated would be needed to accomplish the ambitious goals of the CTSI! This draconian budget reduction created a serious problem of viability for the entire structure, since Indiana CTSI was designed as an interrelated network of painstakingly designed individual programs, each of which was critical for the optimal performance of the entire enterprise. There were important reasons why this complex structure needed to be maintained as a whole to be optimally functional. If we implemented draconian cuts in any single element of the center infrastructure, other program elements could become dysfunctional.

A reduction in size and scope by half would essentially have crippled the CTSI's ability to innovate and make fundamental cultural changes. If we expected scientists in their particular organizational niches (disciplinary and/or depart-mental) to engage in transdisciplinary or interdisciplinary team science (the organizational "culture change" we sought), we would need to have adequate resources to support them in this new endeavor. Absent these resources, the CTSI would have been reduced to barely supporting the existing infrastructure of limited training programs and hospital-based research resources, thus defeat-ing the whole mission of building a statewide biomedical research and training infrastructure.

As noted before, the process of developing the Indiana CTSI took a full year. This unprecedented level of participation by members of diverse schools from IU and PU, and non-academic communities, provided the rich material from which the concept, framework, and proposed activities of the Indiana CTSI were developed; it had also set high expectations for future transformations among all the stakeholders. To say that all the energy, enthusiasm and commitment to reform from the state biomedical research community needed to be curtailed due to budget cuts would have been a tragic loss of opportunity.

Even with a fully funded NIH budget, the resources of the proposed I-CTSI were not large enough by themselves to create a cross-institutional infrastruc-ture. What it did provide was "seed investments" to engage multiple entities to work together, learn best practices from one another, and "nudge" them toward delivering novel translational results. Without the initial stimulus of seed invest-ments, these parties would have been unlikely to make available the protected time, funding incentives and other institutionally valued rewards to work together. Another long-term key challenge raised by the reduction in funding was the potential for failure in applying for continuation funding after the first five years of the CTSA award. In order to remain competitive with other funded CTSAs (some of them receiving as much as three times the total dollar amount awarded to Indiana) and ensure that our federal funding would be renewed in 2013, we would have to accomplish all of our proposed milestones in the current grant, while also needing to demonstrate even greater levels of innovation than initially proposed. Reducing the scope of our goals would seriously compromise Indiana's competitiveness when we went back to the NIH in 2013 to renew this grant along with the other national applicants.

After I overcame my initial shock at the funding shortfall and began to meet with program directors and key stakeholders, I repeatedly heard the same com-ment: "A major reduction in scope will essentially make our program ineffective." As a result, we desperately needed to restore the program budgets to a more manageable scale of reduction – perhaps an average of 15% for the enterprise to get going. For this level of support, I wagered we could challenge each of the programs to deliver fully on the goals they stated within the grant proposal. I explored several options to raise more funds including the Fairbanks Foundation that had pledged its support to the vision of the Indiana CTSI. They had not specifically committed any funds but were keen to enhance the research infrastructure for Indiana, especially in the area of informatics and biobanking. Several meetings with Mr. Len Betley and the Fairbanks leadership quickly resulted in a grant that would provide approximately $700 000 per year for the first four years of the CTSI initiative. This extraordinary gift enabled us to bring every program up to at least 85% of their initial budgets, thus making the vision of the Institute feasible. The first major crisis for the Indiana CTSI was averted by one of its own community partners!

State of the Institute: Three Years and Growing

Three years since its inauguration, all 16 of the Indiana CTSI programs are fully staffed with at least two years of full operations. Overall, the programs are on target with their modified milestones (some milestones were modified from the original proposal due to budgetary constraints), and have created new projects and programs that were not previously envisioned in the original plan.

Since the CTSI was funded, the school of medicine has been fortunate to receive a $60 million gift from the Lilly Endowment to support a program called the Physician Scientist Initiative (PSI). A significant part of these funds (approximately $6 million) was earmarked to develop a large collection of biological samples that can be made available to Indiana researchers. The Indiana CTSI, through its governance structure and multiple programs, created a new program called Indiana Biobank, and plans to collect about 50 000 genetic samples from patients and controls for general research use.

The Biomedical Informatics Program continues the development of information systems to manage samples, phenotypic electronic medical records, and research data, and to identify possible research subject participants. The Community Health Engagement Program and the Bioethics and Subject Advocacy Program (BSAP) are leading the development of policies and strategies to inform the public of opportunities to participate in and contribute to clinical research studies and to assure that clinical research is being conducted at the highest levels of ethical standards. The Regulatory Knowledge and Support program (RKS) is providing leadership in the development of policies and procedures for operation. The Translational Technologies and Resources program has coordinated the policies of a large number of technology cores across the three universities.

We have made significant progress in our efforts to support research subject recruitment, a goal common among most CTSAs. A Subject Recruitment Office was established using CTSA funding in combination with federal economic stimulus (ARRA, the American Recovery and Reinvestment Act of 2009) supplement dollars. The Program provides feasibility assessment for recruiting specific subject populations and methods to identify available patients at appropriate sites. In October of 2010, ResNet, the largest practice-based research network (PBRN) in Indiana, became part of the Indiana CTSI subject recruitment program. In its 10 years of operation this network has recruited on average two of every three patients it has approached with over 16 000 patients having participated in research studies with which it has been involved, a remarkable record of success in any setting. These numbers are especially noteworthy considering that over half of the participants represent minority and underserved populations. The CTSI also established a Volunteer Research Participant Registry, titled INresearch.org. This registry, led by the Indiana CTSI's Recruitment Office and the Community Health Engagement Program, is open to all Indiana residents and Indiana CTSI-affiliated researchers. One of our major hospital systems, Indiana University Health, is formally promoting this registry to its patients.

The Indiana CTSI has also held three large annual meetings on the Indianapolis campus with national and international speakers. There were several hundred attendees at each of these meetings, with faculty scholars and graduate trainees presenting posters and platform talks about their research projects. We have also established a tradition of annual CTSI retreats at each of the partner institution campuses to continue to engage and educate a wide range of faculty and student investigators in the mission of the CTSI. The Indiana CTSI has an electronic newsletter with information and examples of Indiana CTSI investigator successes, new services, program announcements, and funding opportunities. The newsletter builds on the successful communications strategy represented by the Indiana CTSI "HUB," the Internet-based virtual "front door" providing access to all of its services.

One of the key issues that will facilitate clinical and translational research is the Indiana CTSI's commitment to improve performance in the turnaround of institutional review board submissions, contract negotiations and subject enrollment. We have already helped to substantially improve the process at IU and have outlined future goals as noted in Table 3.1.

TABLE 3.1 Indiana CTSI Performance Goals

Metric	Current (2011)	2012	2013	2014
IRB Approval	58 days	48 days	38 days	<30 days
Confidentiality	~10 days	7 days	<5 working days	<5 working days
Full Contracts	~40 days	32 days	25 days	<21 days

The Indiana CTSI provides strong support for pilot grants. In three years, the Indiana CTSI has made hundreds of pilot grant awards, career awards and other research funding totaling over $13.5 million. The Indiana CTSI has conducted three rounds of a novel Collaboration in Translational Research (CTR) grant program. The purpose of these awards is to foster collaborations among partner institutions such as Indiana, Purdue, and Notre Dame universities to conduct translational research projects that have strong potential to develop into larger, continuing, externally funded research programs. We have implemented a metrics-based semi-annual progress reporting system to assess their effectiveness. Using this data, the Indiana CTSI analyzes the results of pilot funding, focusing on external funding, intellectual property development, and publications in peer-reviewed journals.

The Indiana CTSI has another innovative program called the Project Development Team (PDT) which is designed to enhance multidisciplinary clinical and translational research, by providing investigators access to multidisciplinary research expertise, biostatistics, IRB/regulatory services, nursing support, and pilot funds as a "one-stop shop" for investigators. The PDTs have reviewed a total of over 400 proposals and invested about $2 million in seed funds. Over the last year, investigators who went through the PDT process were successful in obtaining nearly $22 million in external grant funds, resulting in an approximately 11-fold return on investment within two years.

The Indiana CTSI Research Education, Training, and Career Development Program continue to build a successful effort to expand the number of clinical researchers. A new Master of Science in Translational Research degree program (as well as companion Graduate Certificate program) was developed and approved for enrollment in 2011 by the Indiana Higher Education Commission. Over 20 clinician-scientists have been funded for career development (KL2) awards and more than 40 graduate student trainees have been funded for predoctoral (TL1) awards per year. We have developed a summer internship program in clinical research for undergraduate scholars. Each year, the Indiana CTSI summer internship program also provides support and funding for 20 to 25 high school students and 20 medical students to be matched with faculty mentors engaged in real-world clinical or laboratory research.

Overall, a total of 153 milestones are being tracked over the first three years of the grant; a total of 61 were scheduled for completion in the first three years. Among these, 53 (86.9%) have been completed, five are under way, and three have been delayed. For the remaining milestones, 86 were scheduled for initiation in the first three years of the grant. Out of these, 77 (89.5%) were actually initiated in the first three years of the grant, four have been delayed, and five are under consideration for modification due to resource levels or possible change in strategy. Six milestones are not scheduled to be initiated until Year 4 of the grant. This continues to be a remarkable accomplishment given continued resource challenges.

Some Lessons Learned

During the development of the Indiana CTSI, and in the first three years of running the Institute, I have learned some important lessons. Although the context of some may be specific to Indiana, the lessons themselves are likely to be applicable to any transformative science program change within an academic medical center in the US and perhaps elsewhere. I will summarize these below.

- Lead with quick wins. Successful academics and clinician-researchers are highly intelligent, superbly focused, driven individuals who are continuously and instinctively thinking through most interactions at work with a single purpose – furthering "their" agenda, be it a research project, a career development goal, or a service activity. When, as an Institute Director, you are implementing initiatives that are well aligned to enhance these individual agendas, it is very easy. People are excited, volunteer their services and generally become ambassadors for these programs. New pilot grant programs are a classic example of such initiatives. For the successful launch of a new institute, begin by sponsoring a lot of these inherently attractive initiatives in the first year.
- Don't avoid important systemic reforms, but be clear about the need for priorities and favorable preconditions for change. When any CTSI initiative involved activities aimed at enhancing group benefits and improving foundational system efficiencies, but with no immediate advantage to individuals, there was a lot of inertia and procrastination evident among investigators. Dealing with people in these reform initiatives required a lot of cajoling and some "carrot-and-stick" incentives and deterrents. I think one should choose

a few of the most important systems issues to tackle early but expect them to take time to become fully instituted. Finally, if there are initiatives that are critical to improving the institutional infrastructure, but clearly involve steps that might be counter to some group's or individual's particular advantage, they will run into every possible delay in implementation. Successful implementation requires a lot of up-front preparation even before reforms are proposed, and some of them are best done in small, incremental steps.

- Expect to cope with boundaries, turf and tribalism – even after academics are out of their silos. A key barrier that I knew would be difficult to overcome, yet completely underestimated its power, was the issue of institutional, school, and departmental boundaries. Successful research organizations, whether in a university or a small center in a department, are powerful "tribes" in their collective psyche and successful researchers within them are intensely tribal creatures. There is something primeval about these silos and it is perilous to ignore this tribal ethos when planning any new initiative. I haven't yet come across an example where one "tribe" conceded their interest fully in the service of the greater good. I am still hoping to be surprised! The partial successes I had overcoming these barriers have always been by finding a "win-win" formula for the groups involved. I have repeatedly come to use the basic principles of game theory trying to find ways to arrive at the best gains for each of the "players."

- Work to align management and control mechanisms. Another barrier to transformative change in academic medical centers is misalignment of control, power, and authority. These misalignments of authority and other management levers permeate complex academic organizations, are sometimes products of diverse accountability and reporting structures, and may be inevitable in our multi-mission, multi-product matrix organizations. Unfortunately, such misalignments also arise as products of historical, personality-driven, or informal social hierarchies in academe. The latter misalignments are not always easy to identify, realign, or resolve effectively. If misalignments have resulted from complex and poorly thought-through organizational logic, they are somewhat easier to address with process improvement exercises like "lean six sigma." Unfortunately, much of the organizational dysfunction in academia falls into the first category (cults of personality and power) and there may be no simple approaches to address them. I believe this issue will be one of the most recalcitrant problems in transforming academic medical centers to become true engines of entrepreneurship and innovation.

So, what is my best advice to someone in my shoes who is trying to establish and run a CTSI-like organization? First, realize that there is no simple recipe for success. We have managed to accomplish a majority of the goals we have set for the Indiana CTSI to date, suggesting that some things we have done have worked. Reflecting on the areas where we have been successful, the approach that has worked for me can be reduced to three basic rules. The first rule is to explore every major issue that arises from multiple viewpoints and with input from many of the diverse stakeholders. The second rule is to discern and communicate a general stakeholder consensus on the nature of the problem and the best possible win-win approach. Once this consensus is established, the final rule is to maintain absolute transparency in your implementation of a solution, while communicating frequently and widely. I have not always been perfect at following these rules, nor has this approach always been successful, but these three simple guides have worked well in enough multiple situations to offer to others.

References

1. Butler D. Translational research: crossing the valley of death. *Nature*. 2008; **453**(7197): 840–2.
2. Kola I, Landis J. Can the pharmaceutical industry reduce attrition rates? *Nat Rev Drug Discov*. 2004; **3**: 711–15.
3. Zerhouni EA. Translational and clinical science: time for a new vision. *N Engl J Med*. 2005; **353**(15): 1621–3.
4. Heller C, de Melo-Martin I. Clinical and Translational Science Awards: can they increase the efficiency and speed of clinical and translational research? *Acad Med*. 2009; **84**(4): 424–32.
5. Hackshaw A, Farrant H, Bulley S, *et al*. Setting up non-commercial clinical trials takes too long in the UK: findings from a prospective study. *J R Soc Med*. 2008; **101**(6): 299–304.
6. Rosenblum D, Alving B. The role of the clinical and translational science awards program in improving the quality and efficiency of clinical research. *Chest*. 2011; **140**(3): 764–7.
7. Califf RM, Berglund L. Linking scientific discovery and better health for the nation: the first three years of the NIH's Clinical and Translational Science Awards. *Acad Med*. 2010; **85**(3): 457–62.
8. Shekhar A, Denne S, Tierney W, *et al*. A model for engaging public-private partnerships. *Clin Transl Sci*. 2011; **4**(2): 80–3.
9. Chang KC, Overhage JM, Hui SL, *et al*. Enhancing laboratory report contents to improve outpatient management of test results. *J Am Med Inform Assoc*. 2010; **17**(1): 99–103.
10. Kho A, Zafar A, Tierney W. Information technology in PBRNs: the Indiana University Medical Group Research Network (IUMG ResNet) experience. *J Am Board Fam Med*. 2007; **20**(2): 196–203.
11. BioCrossroads report. Available at: www.biocrossroads.com/Documents/Indiana-Life-Sciences-Industry_Report-2002-2010.aspx

4

Sparking and Sustaining the Essential Functions of Research

What Supports Translation of Research into Health Care? Answers from the Group Health Experience

Eric B. Larson, Christine Tachibana, and Edward H. Wagner

Eric Larson's Story of a Success in Science: Being An Advocate for Colleagues

A colleague came into my office saying his research had uncovered an amazing finding that he called "hot." It was that people who were getting narcotic analgesics chronically for non-cancer pain were dying at a faster rate than everybody else and he felt it was a real finding. He'd spent his career researching pain. I said well, gosh, that's very important because we've had this whole movement about better treatment of pain in medical care for decades now. We never thought there'd be this kind of a downside. This was not my own research, but his team had sent it off to a prominent journal and it had come back with a rejection. I thought, boy, why would a paper so important get summarily rejected? He and I chatted, and subsequently went back to the editor and asked the journal to take another look – we think this is important material. Some of the reviews were from individuals who probably were not objective in the way they commented on this paper. The editor ought to be aware that there may be reviewers who – no matter how good the research – would recommend against publication. It's a complicated world in which people's other material interests or just reputational self-interest can affect their views of findings, even from good science. Eventually, the paper went through another round of peer-review and editing and was published. When we knew it was going to be published, we began to work with the Group Health delivery system. Almost simultaneously with the knowledge that this finding was going to be published Group Health began to work on how to address this issue health risk. We knew the kind of narcotics that were being prescribed for non-cancer pain and wondered if the side effects of these drugs were causing people to die more frequently. It was also possible that these drugs were being diverted and used for purposes other than pain control – diversion and subsequent abuse of these prescription opioids being an increasing problem in many communities. Group Health was able to examine prescribing data and begin to look at where these clusters of prescriptions were being written, and the challenges of taking care of these patients from doctors' perspectives. They began to develop policies for pain contracts or other kinds of mechanisms to reduce the amount of ongoing prescribing of the medications. By the time the paper was published, a lot of this work was done. Now, nearly all patients receiving chronic opioids have care plans and high dosing is significantly less frequent. The Group Health CEO gave a presentation about research and practice, featuring the story of this study, at Academy Health. The editor of Health Affairs was in the audience, recognized a good story and next thing you know a paper was written that was eventually published in *Health Affairs*. It's a really exciting moment when you know the kind of research we do makes a difference.

Ed Wagner's Story of a Success in Science: Pushing the Envelope Requires Good Group Process

The foundation, from my perspective, for success in science is good group process. The high spots have been when a bunch of disparate individuals, rooted in diverse disciplines, and from different institutions, reach a point when they are functioning as a team, embrace a common purpose and get some important work done. The first big experience of this kind for me was in the Kaiser Family Foundation's Community Health Promotion grant program. I was relatively new to Seattle at the time and got thrust into a leadership role for that study. We were able to put together just a sensational team of people – Tom Koepsell, Bruce Psaty, Paula Diehr, Ed Perrin, and many others. We weren't really sure what the best approaches would be to evaluate the emerging activities of the program. By having all those intellectual powerhouses thinking together, I think we came up with an extraordinarily creative bit of work that was just an extraordinary learning experience for me. We applied methods of randomization and measurement in all kinds of new ways. We did network analysis with a Harvard sociologist. We adopted all kinds of biometry and other measures of community-based nutrition that had never been employed in grocery stores. We went out of our way to encourage crazy ideas, and we had enough money to do so. It's a luxury you often don't have. We did have enough money and enough FTE [full-time equivalents] per person to enable this to happen. I encouraged this process, doing what I think a good facilitator does, helping people push the envelopes so that you don't just settle for the tried and true … same old same old. The other thing I learned then is the importance of not just spreading responsibility but spreading the rewards. I don't know how many different people had first-authored papers but it was a lot. It was an experience of doing science in a group where everybody's contributing … everybody's learning … everybody is having fun! It was a fascinating experience. It was having all that creative energy around the table which gave everybody a chance to play out some of the dreams you don't very often realize. It was fun.

Sparking and Sustaining the Essential Functions of Research: What Supports Translation of Research into Health Care? Answers from the Group Health Experience

The Case for Translating Research Innovations into Clinical Care

Changes in health care can be perceived as threatening and disruptive. The public reaction in 2010 to President Obama's Patient Protection and Affordable Care Act (PPACA) is a memorable example, but it is not unique. Comprehensive health-care reform proposed by President Clinton was so threatening that it was abandoned. In spite of the political challenges, changes in US health care are inevitable. In 2001, the Institute of Medicine (IOM) reported in *Crossing the*

Quality Chasm[1] that health-care quality, access, value, affordability and safety were at crisis levels. In fact, the US health system has long spent twice as much per capita for care than other industrialized countries, with evidence showing that care and outcomes are not better, and patients are not more satisfied. Market-driven health care has led to unsustainable rises in costs, massive increases in people without access to care, and a failure of the United States to keep up with quality improvements achieved in other countries.[2] The claim that the United States has the best care in the world is no longer tenable. Private and public institutions, including academic health science centers, must work together to reverse the rise in health-care expenditures to sustainable levels.

The good news is that we can do better for less if we make smart decisions about how to allocate our health-care resources – a process compared to thinning instead of clear-cutting a forest.[3] Rather than eliminating entire programs or therapies in an attempt to cut costs, we can choose to meet our health-care challenges by following population-based guidelines based on the most rigorous evidence available, with refinement and improvement as new evidence develops. This makes large-scale clinical research with design, testing, and surveillance in real-world populations particularly urgent. Group Health Cooperative, an integrated health-care and delivery system with an embedded research center, is a model for this type of translational health research. Group Health is a learning health system, defined by Carolyn Clancy, director of the Agency for Healthcare Research and Quality (AHRQ), as a system "in which actionable information is made available to clinicians and patients and in which evidence is continually refined as a byproduct of healthcare delivery."[4] The concept of learning health systems, in which research influences practice and practice influences research, reaches back to US health-care reform ideas of the 1990s[5] and has enjoyed a renaissance since the passage of the PPACA.

Three main factors have facilitated the development of Group Health as a learning health system. The first is close and enduring relationships among its clinical arm, its served community, and its non-proprietary, public-interest research center, Group Health Research Institute (GHRI). Another is strategic use of the advantages and resources that come with being an integrated health-care and coverage system. Finally, Group Health is increasingly employing collaborations and national networking, including with academic health centers, to expand its capabilities and broaden its translational impact.

Innovative, game-changing translational health research is possible when health research centers embedded in health-delivery systems form collaborative networks and work with academic partners. These types of networks are generating datasets with a wealth of clinical and coverage information on diverse populations for large, population-based health studies and analysis of the comparative effectiveness of therapies. Health researchers are developing the expertise to link these databases to biologic data from analysis of biobank samples, including genomic, transcriptomic, proteomic and metabolomic data. In 2009, when Francis Collins became director of the National Institutes of Health, he made these types of studies a priority.[6] Perhaps even more noteworthy was his emphasis that research in health-care delivery systems provides unique opportunities for improved efficiency through comparative effectiveness research, previously called outcomes research, including pragmatic clinical trials.

Health-care change will always be both challenging and promising. Group Health, based in Seattle, is recognized for more than 60 years of disruptive innovation in health care. Many of the changes it has implemented – ranging from group practice in the 1940s to broad-based *Chlamydia* screening in the 1990s – are now so common that we almost forget that such things were once rare. Academic health science centers have been vital to these advances. Evidence supporting *Chlamydia* screening came from collaborative research between Group Health and the University of Washington (UW), which have a long history of partnership and, in fact, have grown up together. The UW medical school opened the same year as Group Health, also over objections from the medical establishment, which feared a surplus of physicians. Over the decades, Group Health and its research programs have developed a variety of ongoing research affiliations with the UW.

Becoming a learning health system with mutually beneficial, productive connections to academic partners and other health systems is challenging and it doesn't happen automatically. Communication between research and delivery is a constant work in progress, with continuous improvement as the operating principle. Nonetheless, the Group Health experience is informative in an exploration of the organizational elements of learning health systems on a national scale, and this model could provide solutions to our health-care problems.[7] From this perspective, we present our journey toward effective translational research by focusing on our development as a high-performing learning health system.

Translation Begins with a Research Commitment and a Culture of Change

The founding of Group Health was rooted in change[8–10] (*see* Figure 4.1). Created as Group Health Cooperative in 1947, it offered the radical option of prepaid care from a group of doctors employed by the cooperative, back when the only game

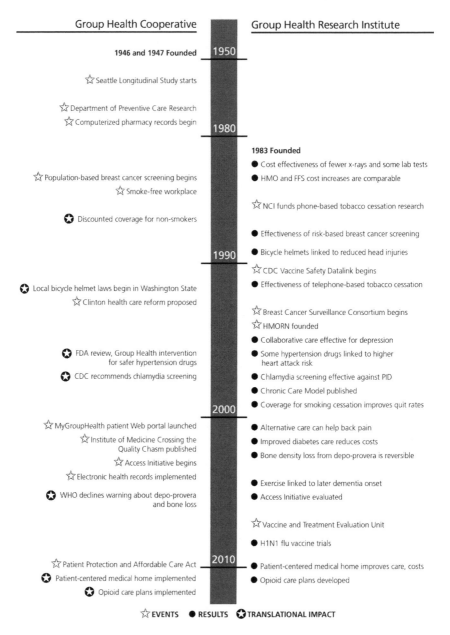

FIGURE 4.1 Group Health and Group Health Research Institute Timeline (preliminary version)

in town was fee-for-service medicine from private hospitals and individual physicians. The founders faced considerable opposition from established practitioners and Seattle hospitals; their survival in an openly hostile environment is chronicled in Paul David Starr's *The Social Transformation of American Medicine*.[11] The consumer-governed organization persisted in introducing group practice, prepaid health coverage, and other innovations, and in 2011 had more than 650,000 members in an integrated care and coverage system. HealthPartners of Minnesota and Group Health are the country's only large, consumer-governed, non-profit health systems. Even as the prevailing approaches to health-care delivery have changed, Group Health has maintained the goal of improving health-care quality while exploring ways to safely contain costs.

Research has always been in the Group Health mission. The preamble of the Group Health Cooperative bylaws, written in 1946, includes support for "projects in the interest of public health" and special attention to preventive medicine. In 1956, the first Group Health research project was initiated under the leadership of Werner Schaie, then a UW graduate student. The Seattle Longitudinal Study on aging is still collecting data on Group Health members and is likely the longest continuous study of aging in the United States.[12] In the 1970s, Group Health began addressing basic issues related to the ethical conduct of research: patient privacy, access to medical records, and informed consent. This era also saw nascent efforts to implement evidence-based standards of practice and protocols while balancing the need for individualized patient care and promoting ongoing patient–provider relationships.

Group Health was also an early adopter of computerized data systems, an important resource for both management and research. In the 1970s, it began computerizing pharmacy records. The resulting database captures the vast majority of member prescription fills, making it particularly valuable for research on pharmacoepidemiology, adherence to medication recommendations, variations in prescribing practices, and other pharmacy-related topics. Stand-alone electronic databases also hold computerized laboratory, admission, discharge, and transfer records, and registries for vaccine and preventive care. In fact, one reason that integrated health systems with stable enrollments such as Group Health are ideal research settings is their access to data on large populations, which facilitates population-based analysis and longitudinal studies. In addition, learning health systems such as Group Health have been leaders in health information technology (IT) with innovations such as development of electronic health records (EHRs), patient Web portals with secure messaging that facilitates doctor–patient communication, and online tools to manage chronic illness. The Group Health patient Web portal allows patients to see parts of their own medical records, communicate with physicians and other providers online, and, since 2011, access these resources through a mobile phone application.

In its early development, Group Health did not have a formal research group to take advantage of the accumulating comprehensive, non-proprietary clinical data on its members. In 1969, the Group Health Research Department was established, led by Richard Handschin, and in 1975, the Department of Preventive Care Research was founded with Robert S. Thompson as its leader. Research activities were not coordinated, but independently conducted by investigators, most of whom were based in academic institutions. In 1981, Gail Warden became the Chief Executive Officer of Group Health. Under his guidance, in 1983, GHRI was founded under its original name, the Center for Health Studies.[9] Ed Wagner was brought in to head the new research center, and with investigator Michael Von Korff, Thompson and a few other stalwarts, formed the nucleus of a group that established the collegial and ambitious culture that endures today.

Partnerships with the UW and the Fred Hutchinson Cancer Research Center (FHCRC) were clearly mutually beneficial and actively promoted by Gilbert S. Omenn, then Dean of the UW School of Public Health; Maureen Henderson, then head of FHCRC's Cancer Prevention Research Program; and other senior faculty. In GHRI's early years, when its faculty consisted of a handful of relatively young investigators, collaborations with senior investigators based at the UW and the FHCRC through large center grants helped build a financial and scientific foundation, eventually cemented with formal affiliation agreements. Nonetheless, in spite of joint faculty appointments and other institutional measures, tensions have occasionally and perhaps inevitably developed, especially as GHRI matured and grew. As it sought to solidify its own funding base, competition over funding was occasionally an issue with its academic partners. However, many of the research collaborations developed in the early years have endured, and GHRI's population and data are a major and sometimes primary research source for UW and FHCRC investigators in cancer, cardiovascular disease, mental health, infectious disease, Alzheimer's disease, geriatric care, and other areas.[13-16] Active involvement with the UW and FHCRC continues. For example, UW graduate students and research fellows such as Robert Wood Johnson (RWJ) Clinical Scholars and trainees at the UW Institute of Translational Health Sciences (the UW's Clinical and Translational Science Awards program) have found GHRI an attractive place for their research. In addition to enhancing the intellectual climate, they provide a steady stream of talented candidates for new faculty positions.

By 2011, GHRI, located in Seattle, had grown to more than 300 employees including 60 faculty members, most with UW joint appointments. GHRI also contains the Center for Community Health and Evaluation, which designs and evaluates health-promoting programs across the country; the Group Health Department of Preventive Care, which is part of Group Health Physicians and provides a link to the clinical practice group; and the MacColl Center for Health Care Innovation, which develops, tests and disseminates strategies that improve health-care quality.

The work of GHRI is aligned with the fundamental principles of the health system in which it is embedded, and we believe this is crucial to its translational successes. GHRI reflects two Group Health priorities: research to improve the quality of health and health care, and a mission to serve the community as a not-for-profit health-care organization. In addition, GHRI was intended from the beginning to contribute to the larger American health system, conducting independent, non-proprietary public interest research, not as a Group Health think tank, but as an open-source health research institute. The relationship between Group Health and its research organization is still evolving but is grounded in a common mission of transforming health and health care through research and innovations in clinical practice and health-care delivery. Our advantage in moving toward this goal is our ability to study populations receiving comprehensive care in integrated delivery systems. An integrated system means that researchers have access to clinical, cost and claims data, expanding the resources for cost-effectiveness research. On the delivery side, being responsible for both care and coverage gives Group Health a strong incentive to safely control costs – an issue that is a high priority with national policy makers and funding agencies.

Translation Benefits from Health System, Researcher, and Community Connections

Before the advent of GHRI, most research using Group Health data was conducted by non-Group Health researchers, typically scientists at major US universities for whom Group Health was just a place that collected data for their scientific observations.[17] Outside researchers can perform capable analyses that yield interesting results, but these types of studies are unconnected to the people who provide the data and are disengaged from the health system that serves them. This is not optimal for either research or translation.

Without a connection to the health system, scientists might pursue questions that are not aligned with the goals of the health system. They do not have an in-depth understanding of the community from which the data came, the context in which the data were collected, or optimal familiarity with the data or the tools for analyzing the particular datasets. Clinical data have unique features such as health system-specific coding and other characteristics influenced by local factors such as changes in health-system policy. These can cause problems for scientists who are using the data without understanding the health-care system, its history and its policies. In short, outside researchers do not understand the nuances of the data that might affect how it should be mined, processed, and interpreted.

For translation, researchers who are not connected to the health system and its members who provided the data are limited in the impact their findings can have on clinical practice. Doctors might not learn of results that are relevant for their patients until they are published in medical journals, often years after completion of a study in which they participated. Without a link to a health system that is involved in the study and will be moving relevant findings into practice, researchers are cut off from valuable translational guidance from clinicians. The practice of exporting large amounts of data for outside research projects without close collaboration of Group Health staff was a concern in the early days of GHRI, and led to at least one example of poorly executed translational science.

In 1981, a study by outside researchers using Group Health data showed a possible connection between vaginal spermicides, birth defects and spontaneous abortions.[17] The study design was criticized by an FDA expert panel and investigators not involved in the study. Richard Watkins, a GHRI investigator and co-author, examined some of the medical records used in the study more closely and found evidence that the presumption of spermicide use in women whose infants had birth defects was faulty. Specifically, a number of these infants appeared to be the result of planned pregnancies, suggesting spermicides were not used.[18] Subsequent studies by other researchers did not support the original findings.[19] In the original study, the results were described as tentative. However, their publication was controversial, and the public received confusing and ultimately inaccurate information. We believe that scientists who partner with a health-care delivery system on study design, data collection, and analysis are likely to consider the translational impact their findings will have on the patients who are contributing data. Although this type of collaboration does not guarantee good study design and accurate interpretation, researchers in a learning health system are more aware of the context of their work than researchers who merely import data from a health system to which they have no connection.

The translational advantages of a research institute with a close relationship to a health system were clear soon after the founding of GHRI (*see* Table 4.1). An early example of a study that influenced health care within the system and eventually nationwide was the 1983 publication of Group Health research showing the cost-effectiveness of a Group Health campaign to reduce unnecessary chest x-rays and certain lab tests.[20] Another example came in 1985, when Group Health established the nation's first population-based breast cancer screening program, supported by federal funding. Thompson realized that the program was an opportunity for Group Health investigators to study the risks, benefits and harms of screening.[21] His team's findings contributed to widespread insurance coverage for breast screening and led to risk-based strategies to improve screening outcomes, as well as ongoing research analyzing the effectiveness of screening for breast and other cancers. This remains a major research area at GHRI. Since 1994, Group Health has been a member of the Breast Cancer Surveillance Consortium, funded by the National Cancer Institute, which links seven mammography registries at academic and health research institutes nationwide for collaborative research on breast screening effectiveness. GHRI serves as the consortium's Statistical Coordinating Center with Diana Miglioretti as principal investigator.

TABLE 4.1 Selected Group Health Research Institute Translational Highlights

Program and Selected Projects	Examples of Translational Impact	Related References
Aging and Geriatrics		
Seattle Longitudinal Study (1956–)	Cognitive training positively affects function; health, environment and personality factors affect risk of cognitive decline. Results shape national efforts on healthy aging.	52
Alzheimer's Disease Patient Registry (1986–2000), Adult Changes in Thought, ACT (1994–)	Evidence for beneficial behaviors and clinical practices for healthy aging, including delaying dementia. Leads to Group Health patient resources on preventive care, exercise, smart eating, maintaining memory, chronic condition care.	14, 47, 53–57
Exercise and aging	Exercise programs reduce risk of falls and fractures. Group Health's Medicare Advantage care covers senior exercise programs.	58–60
Alternate Approaches to Healing		
Complementary and alternative medicine for back pain	Yoga, acupuncture, and massage can be effective for back pain. National guidelines recommend these therapies for back pain and Group Health covers massage for certain types of pain and offers complementary therapy discounts.	61–63
Herbal alternatives for menopause symptoms	Some herbal treatments are not effective for menopause symptoms. Findings incorporated into Group Health patient information.	64

(continued)

Program and Selected Projects	Examples of Translational Impact	Related References
Behavior Change		
Smoking cessation	Effectiveness and cost of telephone-based tobacco cessation counseling and integrated phone + Web programs. Effectiveness and safety of drugs. Free & Clear (Alere Wellbeing) established nationwide. Results change Group Health medication policies and program coverage.	22, 25, 65–67
Bicycle helmets and head injuries	Helmets are effective at preventing head injuries and promoting helmet use is cost-effective. Helmet use increases nationwide.	68, 69
Home blood pressure monitoring (e-BP)	Web-based at-home blood pressure monitoring helps control hypertension. Testing and piloting moves to communities.	51
Weight loss	Interventions in real-life situations (families and workplaces). Development of practical weight control interventions.	70, 71
Biostatistics		
Statistical support for networks	Statistical methods development for the Breast Cancer Surveillance Consortium, Cancer Intervention and Surveillance Modeling Network (CISNET) for colorectal cancer, Centers for Disease Control and Prevention's National Vaccine Safety Datalink project and Food and Drug Administration's Sentinel Initiative. Methods used nationally in safety and effectiveness research.	72–78
Cancer Control		
Population-based breast cancer screening	Early study results show cost-effectiveness, leading to acceptance of insurance coverage for risk-based breast cancer screening. Ongoing research explores screening safety and effectiveness with findings influencing national guidelines.	21, 79–85
Multisite studies through networks: Breast Cancer Surveillance Consortium (1994–), Cancer Biomedical Informatics Grid (caBIG), the Cancer Care Outcomes Research and Surveillance (CanCORS) Consortium, the Cancer Intervention and Surveillance Modeling Network (CISNET, 2000–), and the Cancer Research Network (CRN, 1999–)	Cancer research on etiology, prevention, detection, treatment, survivorship, clinical care, health services and costs, and translational and implementation science using diverse population-based data and in collaboration with national networks. Projects include breast, lung, colorectal, ovarian, prostate, pancreatic cancer, and myeloma, among others for pediatric and adult populations. Results influence local policies and national guidelines.	86–90

Program and Selected Projects	Examples of Translational Impact	Related References
Cardiovascular Health		
Links between heart disease, lifestyle, genetics, medication use	New ways to monitor and treat heart disease and comprehensive analysis of multiple risk factors. Clinical awareness of patient risk factors increases at Group Health and nationally.	91, 92
Safety of drugs for chronic conditions	Some hypertension medications linked to higher heart attack risk. Leads to additional trials, Food and Drug Administration review, and an intervention at Group Health motivating changes to safer drug alternatives.	15, 27, 28
Child and Adolescent Health		
Healthy families and preventive care	Children have specific preventive care needs. Studies on boosting parenting skills, enhancing safety and improving care for chronic conditions such as asthma and depression. Interventions developed to encourage lifelong healthy behavior.	93–95
Improving health care for disadvantaged youth	Cultural competence improves youth care. Impact on research at GHRI and elsewhere on obesity, asthma and other conditions.	96
Chronic Illness Management		
Chronic care model	Model for team-based, patient-centered care improves management of diabetes and other chronic conditions. National implementation through MacColl Center and Robert Wood Johnson-funded Improving Chronic Illness Care.	36, 37, 38, 97
Health Informatics		
Secure websites for patients and providers	Patient-focused health IT assists communication and streamlines clinical practice. MyGroupHealth has health-risk assessment profiles, electronic health records, and other health IT used in the patient-centered medical home.	98
Health Services and Economics		
Studies on health care and economics	Health promotion programs (e.g. smoking cessation) are an effective use of health-care dollars. Findings comparing fee-for-service and Group Health model inform national health-care decisions.	25, 39, 99, 100
Patient-centered medical home	Clinical care model that emphasizes preventive care and chronic disease management, improves collaboration and communication among medical team members, and gives patients greater access. Implemented at Group Health medical centers.	39–43

(continued)

Program and Selected Projects	Examples of Translational Impact	Related References
Immunization and Infectious Disease		
Primary care and AIDS	Primary care management increases survival. Leads to improved care for AIDS patients.	101
Vaccine safety datalink (1990–)	Post-market surveillance of vaccines. Results improve detection of vaccine effectiveness and adverse events.	102
Vaccine and treatment evaluation unit (2007–)	Clinical trials of nationally used vaccines and therapies including flu vaccines. Results disseminated through the National Institute of Allergy and Infectious Diseases.	103
Vaccine hesitancy	Study and intervention features developed. Pilot programs launched to address parent concerns about vaccination.	104
Medication Use and Patient Safety		
Centers for Education and Research on Therapeutics (CERTS)	Studies to optimize safe use of medication and medical products funded by the Agency for Healthcare Research and Quality working with the Food and Drug Administration. Dissemination through the Health Maintenance Organization (HMO) Research Network.	105
Opioid safety	Risk of overdose linked to higher doses. Group Health initiates primary care-based individualized patient care plans to standardize opioid use for chronic non-cancer pain.	29, 30
Mental Health		
Depression and mood disorders	New models for evidence-based patient-centered and collaborative care. At Group Health, individualized depression programs use new communication technology and are integrated with primary care.	106
Mental health care management	Simple, inexpensive care options (team-based primary care, telephone-based treatment) can improve mood disorders and treatment adherence. Findings integral to chronic care and patient-centered care models. Dissemination through national and international advisory boards.	13, 107, 108
Obesity		
Cost-effectiveness and safety of obesity treatments	Multipronged analysis of intervention programs and shared decision making for bariatric surgery. Results used to design optimal research and implementation methods for obesity treatment. Group Health implements shared decision-making patient aids.	109

Program and Selected Projects	Examples of Translational Impact	Related References
Preventive Medicine		
Department of Preventive Care	Health promotion in clinical settings and investigations of surveillance systems and screening tests through a subspecialty in Group Health's medical staff. Physician-scientists conduct studies and develop innovations in care. Translation through collaboration with Group Health clinical quality-improvement activities.	110–112
Women's Health		
Osteoporosis and bone health	Identification of factors that affect bone health (diet, hormone therapy, oral contraceptive use). Findings influence global health guidelines.	113, 114
Menopause symptoms	Rigorous analysis of the effectiveness of alternative treatments. Evidence-based information available for Group Health members.	64
Chlamydia screening	Results on *Chlamydia* screening for at-risk women and pelvic inflammatory disease risk provide evidence for national guidelines.	33, 115

Also in 1985, Group Health began a collaborative research and intervention effort on telephone-based counseling for smoking cessation, initially funded by the National Cancer Institute. Group Health's Center for Health Promotion provided the staff to implement the intervention and GHRI investigators collaborated in the randomized evaluation.[22] GHRI research demonstrated the effectiveness of the implementation[23,24] and the increased effectiveness associated with making smoking cessation services a covered benefit.[25] In 2005, the Center for Health Promotion became the independent commercial tobacco cessation program Free & Clear, Inc. GHRI investigators continue to work with Free & Clear (renamed Alere Wellbeing in 2011) to use telephone-based counseling as a cost-effective method for providing a large population with behavior change interventions.

The Free & Clear initiative highlights several elements that are important for successful health research translation. One is that projects must be closely aligned with health-care system goals – Group Health was one of the first smoke-free workplaces in the country and continues to aggressively promote tobacco cessation in its members and staff. Another is that effective interventions are developed and refined over time, supported by evidence, through many rounds of collaborative work. The Free & Clear self-help intervention has required a concerted and long-term effort by research teams, working with health delivery experts and users, all of whom are necessary for the program's success. This underscores the importance in a translational research project of long-term relationships between partners with diverse expertise, but a common objective.

Research in learning health systems has several features that facilitate national and global implementation. Studies often focus on current major public health issues, and interventions such as telephone-based counseling that are designed to be practical and relatively inexpensive. For example, in 1989, research at GHRI on the effectiveness of bike helmets on preventing cyclists' brain injuries accelerated use of helmets nationwide. Annual traumatic brain injury deaths from cycling in US children aged 5–14 decreased from about 12 per million in 1988 to less than 4 per million in 1998.[26]

A 1995 population-based, case-control study and resulting intervention at Group Health illustrates the translational efficiency that is possible in a learning health system in collaboration with an academic health science center. Bruce Psaty and UW colleagues found that use of short-acting calcium channel blockers such as nifedipine in hypertensive patients is associated with an increased risk of heart attack.[27] This led to a 1996 US FDA recommendation to discourage use of nifedipine for treating high blood pressure. A few months later, Group Health began providing physicians with a summary of evidence about nifedipine, current guidelines about hypertension medication, and patient letters to distribute, advising either a new medication or a physician visit. In a follow-up study of the intervention, Psaty and colleagues found that almost 80% of patients taking short-acting nifedipine had discontinued use within 6 months.[28] Within a year of publication, evidence from a Group Health-UW study influenced national recommendations and led to safer drug use in its member population.

A more recent example of a learning health system using a practical intervention to confront a national health problem comes from a group led by GHRI's Michael Von Korff.[29] First, the team showed that opioid prescriptions for non-cancer chronic pain were increasing at Group Health and other health systems in the United States at the same time that overdoses involving prescribed opioids were rising. Fatal overdoses tripled nationally between 1999 and 2006 to almost 14 000 annual deaths – more than cocaine and heroin overdoses combined. As a result of this and other findings, Group Health began a primary care-based initiative in 2010, working with clinical staff to create care plans for patients who receive opioids for 90 days or longer. Involvement and education of both patients and providers are crucial elements of the initiative, which resulted in care plans for 85% of the target population within 9 months.[30] The strategy, which is currently being evaluated, preceded a 2011 US nationwide action plan to reduce prescription drug abuse. The results demonstrate how a learning health-care system – which facilitates the active involvement of clinical administrators and staff in designing and carrying out studies – can conduct translational research that might be impossible in other settings. Feedback from the care delivery system and input from patients informs interventions based on study results, easing implementation and acceptance by practitioners.

The history of Group Health also contains examples of translational research challenges that we have been slow to address, or for which we are still searching for the best approach. In 1985, investigators working with Group Health published work showing that cost increases at HMOs like Group Health were similar to the fee-for-service sector.[31] Even today, the rate of rise in health-care costs is not appreciably different at Group Health compared to other providers, although Group Health does provide more comprehensive care and benefits. After 27 years, Group Health continues to find that the full value of an integrated delivery system has not yet been achieved and cost savings do not always follow translational successes. In addition, like all research programs, GHRI has projects that have yielded results likely to improve care, but have been slow or even failed to reach patients. An example is a study from the 1990s showing the value of shared decision making,[32] which only achieved follow-up field testing, evaluation, and dissemination beginning in 2009.

Translation is Facilitated by Teamwork: Research Partnerships

To speed the transformation of health-care delivery, Group Health is increasingly looking to partnerships, collaborations, and networks. These have always been a part of GHRI; the first director, Ed Wagner, cultivated relationships with the nearby UW academic health science center and FHCRC and encouraged faculty to establish collaborations. Academic departments, especially in the areas of biostatistics, epidemiology, health services, and social sciences are ready-made partners for learning health systems. They often have faculty who have expertise in population-based research, but lack access to the extensive data of a health system with a focus on health IT, such as Group Health. Faculty at academic institutions can contribute leading-edge expertise in research methods, for example in population sciences, human biology, and clinical specialties; and they have infrastructure and resources such as wet labs that are often lacking in research centers within health systems.

For academic researchers, the connection to a learning health system such as Group Health provides a conduit to moving results into practice. A good example is the collaboration of Delia Scholes and her GHRI colleagues with Walter Stamm and his infectious disease group at UW. Among other accomplishments, in the 1990s this collaboration discovered the importance of *Chlamydia* as a cause of sexually transmitted disease, especially pelvic inflammatory disease, which can lead to infertility and other complications.[33] This research is generally credited with forming the evidence base that changed national medical practice to make screening for *Chlamydia* routine for sexually active women.

Also in the 1990s, in an example of early networking, Group Health became part of the collaborative Vaccine Safety Datalink (VSD) of the Centers for Disease Control and Prevention (CDC). In 2005, the VSD was collecting data on about 2% of the US population. Participation of GHRI researchers led to the ability to work with Group Health data in a local "data warehouse" while combining it with clinical data from other sites. VSD work has been groundbreaking in protecting patient confidentiality, for example through compliance with the 1996 Health Insurance Portability and Accountability Act (HIPAA), while making data available for research. The VSD demonstrates the power of national data linking, as a large population provides the possibility of identifying rare events associated with vaccines. Results with a national impact include contributing timely information on the safety of new vaccines and developing evidence in areas of public controversy over such concerns as mercury-based preservatives in vaccines[34] and claims about a relationship between childhood immunization and autism.[35] In these prominent cases, this capability for surveillance helped to allay public worries about vaccination, working against groups whose fears about vaccine safety can lack scientific rigor.

As an outgrowth of GHRI's contribution to vaccine safety, a group led by Lisa Jackson was selected after competitive review by the National Institute of Allergy and Infectious Diseases as a US center to investigate vaccine effectiveness. Working with partners at Seattle Children's Hospital, the UW and FHCRC, GHRI is now one of eight NIH-funded Vaccine and Treatment Evaluation Units in the country that conduct field clinical trials on new or modified vaccines for infectious disease. GHRI was one of the first programs to administer the swine flu vaccine in the United States during 2009 trials – at a time when rigorous trials needed to be performed quickly because of a predicted global epidemic.

Translational Research is Facilitated by Teamwork: The Collaborative Care Example

A theme in these examples is a long-term focus on population health, with research conducted through multidisciplinary teams whose members come from local and national academic organizations, the health-care delivery system, patient groups, and public and private funding agencies (*see* Figure 4.2). This increasingly connected organizational model is important because translational research is not a one-time transfer of information from research institute to clinic, but an ongoing conversation between researchers, funders, and the community. In this type of relationship, research results that improve health care and the patient experience can have a ripple effect, influencing other research projects and clinical practices. Research informs practice and practice informs research in a cycle analogous to the continuous improvement in the quality-control method "Plan, Do, Check, Adjust" (PDCA).

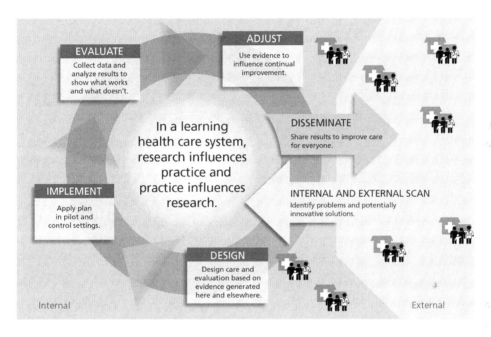

FIGURE 4.2 Learning Health System Model

The organizational benefits of this cycle are seen in improvements at Group Health in common chronic disease treatment, a major research area for many decades. Facing projections of growing chronic illnesses in the United States and worldwide, with many people having multiple conditions, Group Health researchers began a series of trials and observational studies to learn more about the needs of people with chronic diseases such as diabetes, asthma, and cardiovascular disease, to develop ways to more effectively manage their conditions in everyday community settings. The early studies led to observations of shortcomings in care as well as opportunities for improvement. Many of these studies were cited in the influential and inspirational IOM *Crossing the Quality Chasm* report.[1]

From 1992, much of the GHRI work to improve management of common chronic illnesses has been through the MacColl Center for Health Care Innovation. GHRI researchers have been converting chronic care from a reactive response by busy practitioners to proactive management by teams that empower patients who are trained to manage and monitor their own conditions. This team-based, patient-centered chronic care model (CCM) grew out of a series of studies predominantly led by Ed Wagner, David McCulloch, Brian Austin, Michael Von Korff, and others.[36–38] Their work received important, long-term stimulus from the RWJ Foundation, which funded GHRI's MacColl Center for more than 10 years as the national office for the Improving Chronic Illness Care (ICIC), one of RWJ's signature programs. ICIC used CCM principles to lay the groundwork for other projects that address the challenge of long-term, effective management of conditions that are a constant and lifelong concern for affected patients.

The CCM is a prime example of the multidirectional benefit that can occur in a learning health system. Group Health's patient-centered medical home (PCMH) model draws on the CCM and Group Health's efforts in health informatics, among other influences. The PCMH shows how health-care changes are supported by a long-term commitment to evidence-based improvement and continuous cycles of PDCA. In 2002, based on findings that patients needed convenient, patient-centered access to their physicians, and to dispel the misperception that managed care meant barriers to access, Group Health's care delivery team launched the Access Initiative to redesign primary care. This increased the availability of same-day appointments; allowed patient self-referral to specialists; and through a newly launched, secure patient Web portal (MyGroupHealth), encouraged patient communication and medical record review over the Internet. Evaluation of the Access Initiative program by GHRI and researchers in the UW Health Services Department showed that the program increased access and patient satisfaction. Unfortunately, the hoped-for improvement in quality did not materialize, continuity of care actually deteriorated, and the redesign had an overwhelming effect on clinical staff workload.[39,40]

Back at the Group Health drawing board, lessons learned from the Access Initiative sensitized leadership to the importance of a system that had effective primary care as its first principle of design. The challenge was achieving the project goals without burning out primary care physicians and their teams. The solution that was developed is based in the CCM, which identifies specific responsibilities across a team of coordinated but diverse health-care providers and includes patients, families, and community resources. Evidence from GHRI studies demonstrated the effectiveness of collaborative care not only for chronic conditions but for the everyday demands of routine primary care. Based on this understanding, Group Health decided in 2005 to pilot the PCMH, a primary care model that addresses the complexity of 21st-century medicine while supporting the principles of good primary care.[41,42] This model was recommended by the major primary care professional organizations of the time.

The Group Health PCMH model builds on the successful features of the Access Initiative that improved patient access while accommodating longer in-person appointment times. This is balanced by smaller patient panels, care management by clinical teams headed by the primary care physician, and increased use of telephone and electronic contact between patients and the health-care team. Additional provider support comes from Web-based technology for patient communication, outreach and follow-up; and system support for patient involvement in chronic illness care. Physicians are scheduled for "desk time" in addition to direct contact with patients. Among other goals, the PCMH strives to promote continuity and to strengthen ongoing patient–physician relationships. This model is feasible in a setting where physicians are paid per patient or by salary instead of by number of visits or procedures, a feature that is a key element in discussions about reforming the US health-care system to shift the focus from volume to effective care. In this way, Group Health's work on the PCMH matches national priorities such as the establishment through the 2010 PPACA of the Patient-Centered Outcomes Research Institute (PCORI) and the Center for Medicare and Medicaid Innovation (CMMI). PCORI supports research to help patients and providers make informed, evidence-based care decisions. CMMI, part of the Center for Medicare and Medicaid Services, evaluates innovative models of health-care payment and delivery for efficiency and effectiveness, with a goal of improving our national health programs.

Analyses of the PCMH in 2009 by GHRI showed that, compared to control clinics, the changes saved money by reducing emergency care and hospitalizations.[43] The analysis also showed improvements in quality, patient experience, and clinician burnout. In 2010, Group Health implemented the PCMH at all 26 of its medical clinics. Evaluation of this project is ongoing. In the meantime, GHRI has become a bellwether and leader in the PCMH movement, which has become an important element in the country's efforts to improve care, contain costs, and increase health-care access. Acting CMMI director Richard J. Gilfillan visited GHRI to learn about the PCMH as an example of a timely evaluation of an intervention that allowed Group Health to make an opportune, evidence-based decision about system-wide implementation. The PCMH is also one of the best examples of how a learning health system can be successful only if it strives for ongoing improvement, with the understanding that this also requires evaluation and adjustment.

Group Health's successful transition to the PCMH model relied heavily on health informatics advances already implemented by our organization. In 2006, when EHRs and Web-based patient communication technology had been sufficiently developed, Group Health launched a personalized health-risk appraisal, The Health Profile, in its online patient records. The Health Profile uses evidence-based, self-reported measures of health risk combined with measures of "stages of change," derived from behavior-change theory, to provide individual recommendations for positive lifestyle changes, such as weight loss. Recommendations are based on regular patient updates and are tailored to the patient's readiness and interest in making changes and are linked to relevant resources. The profile provides a starting point for a dialog between patient and physician, made possible through the continuity of care established through the PCMH. It can also be used for studies that require clinical information that is difficult to obtain through other sources, such as patient-reported health behavior. In this way, it serves as a database for research analogous to GHRI's widely used breast cancer risk database and could be linked to biobanks for personalized medicine research.

National Translation through Networking: HMORN

Our health-care problems are national in scope, so our solutions must be as well. The problems and challenges facing US health care are complex, requiring multidisciplinary input from traditional researchers as well as experts on health-related communication, economics, informatics, and dissemination. As Barbara Alving points out in her foreword to this book, creative collaboration and networking between the public and private sectors, research institutions, universities, and funders can amplify the advantages of each contributor. At the same time, individual partners must have autonomy in conducting health research and implementing findings, since they are in the best position to work with their scientists, clinical staff, and served population. These factors must be considered in establishing collaborations and networks, whether they are of health research organizations or academic research centers.

As an organizational model, the benefits of national networks are greater access to broader scientific expertise and larger and more diverse populations for increased generalizability, statistical power, and ability to detect rare events. As a result, studies that compare different care systems can be performed. In addition, study findings often have a broader impact, as results are shared through national networks. For these reasons, Ed Wagner worked to create the Health Maintenance Organization Research Network (HMORN), of which Group Health is an original member. Founded in 1995, HMORN grew to a consortium of 19 research centers in 2011, including HealthPartners described above, and regional Kaiser Permanente health systems among others across the country. All are non-proprietary, public interest research centers within health-care systems with a commitment to doing science in the public domain.

With its academic collaborators and funding partners, which include the NIH, the AHRQ, the CDC, and private foundations, HMORN hopes to facilitate national translation through enduring, mutually beneficial partnerships. HMORN expands the learning health system to an enterprise with national and international potential to improve care through population-based, delivery system research. Pathbreaking epidemiology and health services research networks resulting from the HMORN include the VSD, the Cancer Research Network (CRN) originally funded by the National Cancer Institute in 1999, and others (*see* Table 4.2).

TABLE 4.2 HMORN-affiliated Research Networks

Project Name	Study Period	Funding Agency	# HMORN Sites	Focus
Vaccine Safety Datalink (VSD)	1990– current	CDC	10	Vaccine effectiveness, outcomes
Cancer Research Network (CRN)	1999– current	NCI	14	Cancer prevention, control, outcomes
Centers for Education and Research in Therapeutics (CERT)	2000– 2011	AHRQ	13	Safety, effectiveness, appropriateness of use of drugs, biologics, devices
Integrated Delivery System Research Network (IDSRN)	2000– 2005	AHRQ	11	Care delivery and research diffusion in integrated health-care systems
National Bioterrorism Surveillance Project	2000– ~2004	CDC	8	Syndromic surveillance methods
Cancer Care and Outcomes Research Surveillance Consortium (CanCORS)	2001– current	NCI	5	Experience of newly diagnosed lung or colorectal cancer patients
Coordinated Clinical Studies Network (CCSN)	2004– 2008	NHLBI	10	Creation of a shared, sustainable infrastructure to facilitate research
Developing Evidence to Improve Decisions about Effectiveness (DEcIDE)-1 Network	2005– current	AHRQ	12	Comparative treatment effectiveness and safety

(continued)

Project Name	Study Period	Funding Agency	# HMORN Sites	Focus
Cardiovascular Research Network (CVRN)	2007– current	NHLBI	14	Cardiovascular disease epidemiology, management, and outcomes
Developing Evidence to Improve Decisions about Effectiveness (DEcIDE)-2 Network	2008– current	AHRQ	14	Comparative treatment effectiveness and safety
Research Program in Medication Use and Outcomes in Pregnancy (MEPREP)	2009– current	FDA	11	Medication exposure during pregnancy and maternal/fetal outcomes using linked data
Mini Sentinel Network (MSN)	2009– current	FDA	13	Development of active surveillance systems for FDA safety monitoring
Accelerating Change and Transformation in Organizations and Networks (ACTION II)	2010– current	AHRQ	14	Practice-based, implementation-oriented, rapid cycle research
Mental Health Research Network (MHRN)	2010– current	NIMH	10	Conduct rapid and efficient effectiveness trials in mental health
Population-based Effectiveness in Asthma and Lung Diseases (PEAL) Network	2010– current	AHRQ ARRA	4	Accelerate comparative effectiveness research in asthma and other lung diseases in diverse populations
Surveillance, Prevention, and Management of Diabetes Mellitus (SUPREME-DM)	2010– current	AHRQ ARRA	12	Study trends in diabetes incidence and prevalence, and diabetes treatment patterns and outcomes
Scalable PArtnership Network (SPAN) for Comparative Effectiveness Research	2010– current	AHRQ ARRA	10	Distributed data network to support CER

CDC, Centers for Disease Control and Prevention; NCI, National Cancer Institute; AHRQ, Agency for Healthcare Research and Quality; NHLBI, National Heart, Lung and Blood Institute; FDA, US Food and Drug Administration; NIMH, National Institute of Mental Health; ARRA, American Recovery and Reinvestment Act

HMORN data management innovations provide an excellent example of a networking organizational model. First, GHRI scientists developed methods to convert data that had been collected for clinical purposes into datasets suitable for research. When GHRI began collaborating with other embedded research centers, differences in data definitions and management practices became apparent. To ease sharing while preserving patient privacy and keeping control of the data in the hands of the people who best understand them, the CRN created the Virtual Data Warehouse (VDW). The VDW standardizes data, and at the same time gives each participating site stewardship over its own resources. Data from multiple sites are combined into datasets as needed for research. This eliminates the need for a single massive database, and allows studies that would not have been possible if conducted by scientists working individually.[44] This organizational model illustrates how each site views its data – not as something that the researchers own, but something they are responsible for – and ensures that use is open source, non-proprietary and in the public interest. Sharing is facilitated but autonomy is maintained.

In addition to providing greater access to data, national consortia like the HMORN have several specific advantages. For example, HMORN members have extensive experience in mining, processing, and interpreting their own data, and sharing information accurately and securely – simply put, researchers in integrated delivery systems know what to do with data derived from ongoing care in their systems. As well, national health research networks increase the types of studies possible. In addition to conducting traditional observational studies, which have been the mainstay of delivery system surveillance research, a health system network has the ability to conduct the types of pragmatic, real-world clinical studies that the IOM, in a 2006 roundtable workshop on evidence-based medicine[45] suggested could benefit translation of research findings into clinical practice. Finally, membership in HMORN care systems is reasonably stable, allowing long-term analysis of the entire picture of the health and health-care experiences of a large, real-world population over time. This includes screening, treatment, prescriptions, and costs. Rather than relying on convenience samples or referral-filtered groups, the HMORN can conduct longitudinal, population-based studies on subjects more representative of their communities. Natural experiments can be particularly valuable for HMORN researchers, when practice changes or simple variability in practice or coverage provide an opportunity to examine effects on outcomes and perform surveillance studies. The network can also conduct randomized controlled trials – both traditional efficacy trials and so-called pragmatic or real-life trials – in community populations, using methods to detect and adjust for non-randomness of participants.

Health research consortia also have the potential to conduct novel health research aimed at individualizing diagnoses and therapies. HMORN sites are already developing ways to securely link data from EHRs and biobanks and are looking to combine local expertise about each site's clinical datasets and samples with the growing genomic, proteomic, and metabolomic databases. Combining this capability with health systems providing everyday ongoing care is an opportunity for national mega-epidemiology studies.

Translation is about Relationships

While expanding its reach nationally through the HMORN, Group Health also works to ensure its research remains locally relevant. We have learned that effective translation is greatly enhanced when relationships between a health research organization and a health delivery system that is committed to evidence-based improvements in health care are bidirectional. As well, both the research and clinical arms must be closely tied to the community. GHRI study participants are typically members of the cooperative health plan, and ideally see their involvement as a partnership between themselves and Group Health. For example, in cohort studies, we aim to create a relationship between participants and researchers that helps participants experience the satisfaction of "giving" to a research effort and understand how their contribution will benefit others.

A 2010 study from the eMERGE network within the HMORN demonstrates the benefits of fostering an ongoing, trust-based relationship with study participants[46] – the kind of relationship that is possible through researchers' connection to a membership-based health plan. Participants in the Group Health Adult Changes in Thought (ACT) study were asked about re-consenting to having their medical and genetic data included anonymously in a federal database. Of respondents, 90% thought it was important to be asked again, even though they had already consented to participation in ACT. Participants said that improving patient care and contributing to knowledge were important factors in the consent decision. They named their relationship with the researchers they were working with as a strong, positive influence. Negative influences were concerns about privacy, and especially use of their data for profit. As a demonstration of the loyalty of the Group Health community, the ACT study has been ongoing with good retention since 1994, and although participants are randomly selected, several are among the original Group Health founders.

A solid relationship between participants who provide clinical data and the research institution collecting the data fulfills an important ethical obligation of good data stewardship. GHRI studies aim to inform participants of study progress and findings as a way of recognizing their contributions to improving health care for everyone. In the best case, participants will have trust and confidence in the research team and its parent institution. From a practical standpoint, this benefits the health system and researchers interested in developing the most robust research, because a good participant-research relationship encourages ongoing participation, avoiding excessive study disenrollment that can threaten study validity.

We have also found that a healthy, mutually beneficial relationship between researchers and participants, developed and maintained over time, improves study enrollment and allows for more robust study designs. For example, the Kame project was a study on aging initiated in 1992 and affiliated with the ACT study. Participants were older Japanese Americans who resided in King County, which includes Seattle. The study benefited from direct community input. Members of the Kame project's Community Advisory Board early on alerted researchers to the community's heightened sensitivity to an everyday census. This was based in the registration of Japanese community members at the start of World War II and their subsequent forced internment – a concern other research projects had failed to appreciate. Researchers developed recruitment materials with this consideration in mind and enjoyed a long-term relationship with the community that continued even after the study ended. To "give back" to the study population, all Kame participants and their family members received a comprehensive summary of the Kame project's results and also a print of a traditional-style original woodcut donated by one of the study's participants.

The longitudinal cohort ACT study, initiated in 1994, follows Group Health participants over age 65 to identify risk factors associated with cognitive decline. Results are returned to the participants in a quarterly newsletter that translates the results of recent research, for example on the benefits of exercise, into health tips about common problems of aging, such as falling or joint aches. Earlier results from Group Health research led to programs like Silver Sneakers and Lifetime Fitness that promote exercise in older persons. Study results also led Group Health and other insurers to include coverage of senior exercise programs as part of the Medicare Advantage program. ACT findings have supported regular exercise to possibly prevent or delay onset of dementia in older persons[47–49] and this has been advanced as a powerful motivator for the behavior change required to achieve regular physical activity.

As with other elements of GHRI studies, community involvement works because it is aligned with Group Health priorities. Rather than simply advancing one-time-only changes with no evaluation or attempt for continuous improvement, learning health systems aim for progressive improvements to health-care quality. This is aided by studies in which trial participants and their families are equal partners with health-care research organizations from the beginning, a concept called community-based participatory research.[50] Patient and family involvement provides momentum and motivation to follow through on study findings, creating a "culture of results" that strives to get results into practice as quickly as possible, according to Maria T. Britto, Director, Center for Innovation in Chronic Disease Care, Cincinnati Children's Hospital.

Members of the public might benefit from learning health systems even if they do not belong to the care system. An example is the innovative Group Health e-BP program, designed to improve treatment of hypertension, which is the most commonly diagnosed condition in primary care but is controlled in only 50% of people with the diagnosis. Elements of the program are at-home self-monitoring of blood pressure with results tracked and reviewed online through Group Health's secure patient portal (MyGroupHealth) by a pharmacist who provides medication and self-management support. Effectiveness was demonstrated in a randomized trial in 2008,[51] which found improved overall blood pressure control, especially among those with poor control before the program. GHRI and the NIH Clinical Translational Science Awards program at the UW funded pilot projects to move e-BP beyond the Group Health system into rural communities in Washington and Idaho.

The e-BP project is an example of the sophisticated translational accomplishments that are possible when a collaboration is based on long-term relationships between learning health systems, funding agencies, and academic health science centers. These partnerships are fruitful when they are based in a shared vision, principles, and expectations. These start with individuals working together on local and regional projects, but can have national impact when successful models are disseminated through networks such as the HMORN. The challenge for both learning health systems and academic centers is fostering an environment in which individuals can flourish across institutional boundaries and tribal loyalties.

Translation Means that Learning Health Systems Evolve

The fundamental principle of a learning health system is to be constantly improving, which makes stating organizational ground rules difficult. Nonetheless, at Group Health, the relationship between GHRI and the health plans' larger organization is trending toward increasing integration. In 2011, the position of Associate Medical Director of Health Services Research and Knowledge Translation was created to strengthen the relationship between GHRI and Group Health operations. GHRI investigator Rob Reid, who led the evaluation of the PCMH, was appointed to the position. Also in 2011, GHRI Executive Director Eric Larson was appointed Vice President for Research at Group Health. These administrative events point to the commitment by Group Health leadership to support a strong, non-proprietary public interest research operation that enjoys a long-term relationship built on learning health system principles that naturally join the research arm and delivery system. Already, these closer ties have facilitated the planning of pilot research projects by GHRI researchers to be conducted at Group Health Medical Centers. To enhance bidirectionality, the Group Health Foundation has launched the Partnership for Innovation program to solicit novel ideas from frontline providers who will work with research faculty and staff to refine projects and produce evaluations. These collaborations will provide leadership with evidence for decisions on the most important step of an innovation: what happens after the research.

Evolution of the HMORN into a truly national learning health system is a possibility, in light of HMORN growth from 13 members in 2004 to 19 members in 2011. A national learning health system will allow population-based research that is informed and guided by community input, and can take advantage of high-throughput systems biology methods. Results, when appropriate, can move more efficiently and quickly into practice and will facilitate more informed decisions by patients and providers. This vision is supported by national leaders, such as NIH Director Francis Collins, who emphasized projects in epidemiology and translational medicine with a goal of advancing more personalized medicine.[6]

The health-care challenges we currently face are complicated by global economic events and the politicization of health-care reform. We believe that now is the time to push for changes in the way we do health-care research. Specifically, we must wring all possible advantages out of the expertise in our academic, government, and research institutions; we must fully explore our resources such as EHRs, databases and the algorithms developed to work with them, and our physical resources such as biobanks. We must work with our human resources such as patients and communities that share our goal of improving health care. In fact, we believe that maintaining a relationship based on mutuality among researchers, providers, and health system members will demonstrate the value of health research and favorably alter public opinion of evidence-based medicine.

In summary, we need to make ongoing national research based in learning health systems a priority. Selected leaders at the NIH and in government understand this vision, but additional senior leadership and policy makers must be convinced of the value of this organizational model. Our experience with translational research has taught us that close relationships among academic health science centers and health-care systems can be a valuable part of this model. These start with long-term collaborative relationships between researchers with mutual scientific interests and goals and a shared commitment to implementing their findings as evidence-based care. Local and regional partnerships benefit from a connection to the same community, and research networks are vital for disseminating successful findings nationwide. Trusting relationships among providers, researchers, funders and communities can help convince governments and the public of the enduring value of this model of health-care improvement.

References

1. Committee on the Quality of Health Care in America, Institute of Medicine of the National Academies, editors. *Crossing the Quality Chasm: a new health system for the 21st century.* Washington, DC: National Academies Press; 2001.
2. Davis K, Schoen C, Schoenbaum SC, *et al. Mirror, Mirror on The Wall: an international update on the comparative performance of American health care.* New York: The Commonwealth Fund; 2007.
3. Welch HG. Should the health care forest be selectively thinned by physicians or clear cut by payers? *Ann Intern Med.* 1991; **115**(3): 223–6.
4. Olsen L, McGinnis JM. *Redesigning the Clinical Effectiveness Research Paradigm: Innovation and Practice-Based Approaches: Workshop Summary 2010.* Available at: www.ncbi.nlm.nih.gov/books/NBK51016/
5. Etheredge LM. A rapid-learning health system. *Health Aff (Millwood).* 2007; **26**(2): w107–18.
6. Collins FS. Research agenda. Opportunities for research and NIH. *Science.* 2010; **327**(5961): 36–7.
7. Larson EB. Group Health Cooperative: one coverage-and-delivery model for accountable care. *N Engl J Med.* 2009; **361**(17): 1620–2.
8. Crowley W. *To Serve the Greatest Number: a history of Group Health Cooperative of Puget Sound.* Seattle, WA: University of Washington Press; 1996.
9. Group Health Research Institute. Group Health Research Institute milestones. Available at: www.grouphealthresearch.org/aboutus/milestones.html
10. Zerhouni EA. Translational and clinical science: time for a new vision. *N Engl J Med.* 2005; **353**(15): 1621–3.
11. Starr P. *The Social Transformation of American Medicine.* New York: Basic Books; 1982.
12. Schaie KW. *Developmental Influences on Adult Intelligence: the Seattle longitudinal study.* New York: Oxford University Press; 2005.
13. Katon W, Von Korff M, Lin E, *et al.* Collaborative management to achieve treatment guidelines. Impact on depression in primary care. *JAMA.* 1995; **273**(13): 1026–31.
14. Kukull WA, Higdon R, Bowen JD, *et al.* Dementia and Alzheimer disease incidence: a prospective cohort study. *Arch Neurol.* 2002; **59**(11): 1737–46.
15. Psaty BM, Koepsell TD, Wagner EH, *et al.* The relative risk of incident coronary heart disease associated with recently stopping the use of beta-blockers. *JAMA.* 1990; **263**(12): 1653–7.
16. Chen CL, Weiss NS, Newcomb P, *et al.* Hormone replacement therapy in relation to breast cancer. *JAMA.* 2002; **287**(6): 734–41.
17. Jick H, Walker AM, Rothman KJ, *et al.* Vaginal spermicides and congenital disorders. *JAMA.* 1981; **245**(13): 1329–32.
18. Watkins RN. Vaginal spermicides and congenital disorders: the validity of a study. *JAMA.* 1986; **256**(22): 3095–6.
19. Louik C, Mitchell AA, Werler MM, *et al.* Maternal exposure to spermicides in relation to certain birth defects. *N Engl J Med.* 1987; **317**(8): 474–8.
20. Thompson RS, Kirz HL, Gold RA. Changes in physician behavior and cost savings associated with organizational recommendations on the use of "routine" chest X rays and multichannel blood tests. *Prev Med.* 1983; **12**(3): 385–96.
21. Thompson R TS, Carter AP, Schnitzer F, *et al.* A risk-based breast cancer screening at Group Health Cooperative of Puget Sound. *HMO Pract.* 1988; **2**: 177–91.

22. Orleans CT, Schoenbach VJ, Wagner EH, *et al.* Self-help quit smoking interventions: effects of self-help materials, social support instructions, and telephone counseling. *J Consult Clin Psychol.* 1991; **59**(3): 439–48.

23. Curry SJ, Wagner EH, Grothaus LC. Evaluation of intrinsic and extrinsic motivation interventions with a self-help smoking cessation program. *J Consult Clin Psychol.* 1991; **59**(2): 318–24.

24. Curry SJ. Self-help interventions for smoking cessation. *J Consult Clin Psychol.* 1993; **61**(5): 790–803.

25. Curry SJ, Grothaus LC, McAfee T, *et al.* Use and cost effectiveness of smoking-cessation services under four insurance plans in a health maintenance organization. *N Engl J Med.* 1998; **339**(10): 673–9.

26. Thompson R. *Transforming Health Care for Preventive Care Services 30 Years of Learning: projections for the future.* Birnbaum Lecture, GroupHealth Research Institute; 2004.

27. Psaty BM, Heckbert SR, Koepsell TD, *et al.* The risk of myocardial infarction associated with antihypertensive drug therapies. *JAMA.* 1995; **274**(8): 620–5.

28. Kaplan RC, Psaty BM, Kriesel D, *et al.* Replacing short-acting nifedipine with alternative medications at a large health maintenance organization. *Am J Hypertens.* 1998; **11**(4 Pt 1): 471–7.

29. Dunn KM, Saunders KW, Rutter CM, *et al.* Opioid prescriptions for chronic pain and overdose: a cohort study. *Ann Intern Med.* 2010; **152**(2): 85–92.

30. Trescott CE, Beck RM, Seelig MD, *et al.* Group Health's initiative to avert opioid misuse and overdose among patients with chronic noncancer pain. *Health Aff (Millwood).* 2011; **30**(8): 1420–4.

31. Newhouse JP, Schwartz WB, Williams AP, *et al.* Are fee-for-service costs increasing faster than HMO costs? *Med Care.* 1985; **23**(8): 960–6.

32. Wagner EH, Barrett P, Barry MJ, *et al.* The effect of a shared decision-making program on rates of surgery for benign prostatic hyperplasia. Pilot results. *Med Care.* 1995; **33**(8): 765–70.

33. Scholes D, Stergachis A, Heidrich FE, *et al.* Prevention of pelvic inflammatory disease by screening for cervical chlamydial infection. *N Engl J Med.* 1996; **334**(21): 1362–6.

34. Thompson WW, Price C, Goodson B, *et al.* Early thimerosal exposure and neuropsychological outcomes at 7 to 10 years. *N Engl J Med.* 2007; **357**(13): 1281–92.

35. Price CS, Thompson WW, Goodson B, *et al.* Prenatal and infant exposure to thimerosal from vaccines and immunoglobulins and risk of autism. *Pediatrics.* 2010; **126**(4): 656–64.

36. Wagner EH, Austin BT, Davis C, *et al.* Improving chronic illness care: translating evidence into action. *Health Aff (Millwood).* 2001; **20**(6): 64–78.

37. Battersby M, Von Korff M, Schaefer J, *et al.* Twelve evidence-based principles for implementing self-management support in primary care. *Jt Comm J Qual Patient Saf.* 2010; **36**(12): 561–70.

38. Wagner EH, Austin BT, Von Korff M. Organizing care for patients with chronic illness. *Milbank Q.* 1996; **74**(4): 511–44.

39. Conrad D, Fishman P, Grembowski D, *et al.* Access intervention in an integrated, prepaid group practice: effects on primary care physician productivity. *Health Serv Res.* 2008; **43**(5 Pt 2): 1888–905.

40. Tufano JT, Ralston JD, Martin DP. Providers' experience with an organizational redesign initiative to promote patient-centered access: a qualitative study. *J Gen Intern Med.* 2008; **23**(11): 1778–83.

41. Reid RJ, Fishman PA, Yu O, *et al.* Patient-centered medical home demonstration: a prospective, quasi-experimental, before and after evaluation. *Am J Manag Care.* 2009; **15**(9): e71–87.

42. Larson EB, Reid R. The patient-centered medical home movement: why now? *JAMA.* 2010; **303**(16): 1644–5.

43. Reid RJ, Coleman K, Johnson EA, *et al.* The group health medical home at year two: cost

savings, higher patient satisfaction, and less burnout for providers. *Health Aff (Millwood)*. 2010; **29**(5): 835–43.

44. Hornbrook MC, Hart G, Ellis JL, *et al.* Building a virtual cancer research organization. *J Natl Cancer Inst Monogr*. 2005; **35**: 12–25.

45. Olsen L, Aisner L, McGinnis JM, editors. *The Learning Healthcare System: Workshop Summary (IOM Roundtable on Evidence-Based Medicine)*. Washington DC: The National Academies Press; 2007.

46. Ludman EJ, Fullerton SM, Spangler L, *et al.* Glad you asked: participants' opinions of re-consent for dbGap data submission. *J Empir Res Hum Res Ethics*. 2010; **5**(3): 9–16.

47. Larson EB, Wang L, Bowen JD, *et al.* Exercise is associated with reduced risk for incident dementia among persons 65 years of age and older. *Ann Intern Med*. 2006; **144**(2): 73–81.

48. Wang L, Larson EB, Bowen JD, *et al.* Performance-based physical function and future dementia in older people. *Arch Intern Med*. 2006; **166**(10): 1115–20.

49. Sonnen JA, Larson EB, Crane PK, *et al.* Pathological correlates of dementia in a longitudinal, population-based sample of aging. *Ann Neurol*. 2007 Oct; **62**(4): 406–13.

50. Schmittdiel JA, Grumbach K, Selby JV. System-based participatory research in health care: an approach for sustainable translational research and quality improvement. *Ann Fam Med*. 2010; **8**(3): 256–9.

51. Green BB, Cook AJ, Ralston JD, *et al.* Effectiveness of home blood pressure monitoring, web communication, and pharmacist care on hypertension control: a randomized controlled trial. *JAMA*. 2008; **299**(24): 2857–67.

52. Schaie KW, Willis SL, Caskie GI. The Seattle longitudinal study: relationship between personality and cognition. *Neuropsychol Dev Cogn B Aging Neuropsychol Cogn*. 2004; **11**(2–3): 304–24.

53. Larson EB. Physical activity for older adults at risk for Alzheimer disease. *JAMA*. 2008; **300**(9): 1077–9.

54. Larson EB, Kukull WA, Teri L, *et al.* University of Washington Alzheimer's Disease Patient Registry (ADPR): 1987–1988. *Aging (Milano)*. 1990; **2**(4): 404–8.

55. Kukull WA, Hinds TR, Schellenberg GD, *et al.* Increased platelet membrane fluidity as a diagnostic marker for Alzheimer's disease: a test in population-based cases and controls. *Neurology*. 1992; **42**(3 Pt 1): 607–14.

56. Kukull WA, Schellenberg GD, Bowen JD, *et al.* Apolipoprotein E in Alzheimer's disease risk and case detection: a case-control study. *J Clin Epidemiol*. 1996; **49**(10): 1143–8.

57. Larson EB, Shadlen MF, Wang L, *et al.* Survival after initial diagnosis of Alzheimer disease. *Ann Intern Med*. 2004; **140**(7): 501–9.

58. Teri L, McCurry SM, Logsdon RG, *et al.* A randomized controlled clinical trial of the Seattle Protocol for Activity in older adults. *J Am Geriatr Soc*. 2011; **59**(7): 1188–96.

59. Buchner DM, Beresford SA, Larson EB, *et al.* Effects of physical activity on health status in older adults. II. Intervention studies. *Annu Rev Public Health*. 1992; **13**: 469–88.

60. Wagner EH, LaCroix AZ, Buchner DM, *et al.* Effects of physical activity on health status in older adults. I. Observational studies. *Annu Rev Public Health*. 1992; **13**: 451–68.

61. Cherkin DC, Sherman KJ, Kahn J, *et al.* A comparison of the effects of 2 types of massage and usual care on chronic low back pain: a randomized, controlled trial. *Ann Intern Med*. 2011; **155**(1): 1–9.

62. Chou R, Qaseem A, Snow V, *et al.* Diagnosis and treatment of low back pain: a joint clinical practice guideline from the American College of Physicians and the American Pain Society. *Ann Intern Med*. 2007; **147**(7): 478–91.

63. Cherkin DC, Eisenberg D, Sherman KJ, *et al.* Randomized trial comparing traditional Chinese medical acupuncture, therapeutic massage, and self-care education for chronic low back pain. *Arch Intern Med*. 2001; **161**(8): 1081–8.

64. Newton KM, Reed SD, LaCroix AZ, *et al.* Treatment of vasomotor symptoms of menopause

with black cohosh, multibotanicals, soy, hormone therapy, or placebo: a randomized trial. *Ann Intern Med*. 2006; **145**(12): 869–79.

65. Swan GE, McAfee T, Curry SJ, *et al*. Effectiveness of bupropion sustained release for smoking cessation in a health care setting: a randomized trial. *Arch Intern Med*. 2003; **163**(19): 2337–44.

66. Swan GE, McClure JB, Jack LM, *et al*. Behavioral counseling and varenicline treatment for smoking cessation. *Am J Prev Med*. 2010; **38**(5): 482–90.

67. McClure JB, Swan GE, Catz SL, *et al*. Smoking outcome by psychiatric history after behavioral and varenicline treatment. *J Subst Abuse Treat*. 2010; **38**(4): 394–402.

68. Thompson DC, Rivara FP, Thompson R. Helmets for preventing head and facial injuries in bicyclists. *Cochrane Database Syst Rev*. 2000(2): CD001855.

69. Thompson RS, Rivara FP, Thompson DC. A case-control study of the effectiveness of bicycle safety helmets. *N Engl J Med*. 1989; **320**(21): 1361–7.

70. Ludman E, Simon GE, Ichikawa LE, *et al*. Does depression reduce the effectiveness of behavioral weight loss treatment? *Behav Med*. 2010; **35**(4): 126–34.

71. Benedict MA, Arterburn D. Worksite-based weight loss programs: a systematic review of recent literature. *Am J Health Promot*. 2008; **22**(6): 408–16.

72. Nelson JC, Bittner RC, Bounds L, *et al*. Compliance with multiple-dose vaccine schedules among older children, adolescents, and adults: results from a vaccine safety datalink study. *Am J Public Health*. 2009; **99**(Suppl 2): S389–97.

73. Knudsen AB, Lansdorp-Vogelaar I, Rutter CM, *et al*. Cost-effectiveness of computed tomographic colonography screening for colorectal cancer in the medicare population. *J Natl Cancer Inst*. 2010; **102**(16): 1238–52.

74. Miglioretti DL, Heagerty PJ. Marginal modeling of multilevel binary data with time-varying covariates. *Biostatistics*. 2004; **5**(3): 381–98.

75. Rutter CM, Zaslavsky AM, Feuer EJ. Dynamic microsimulation models for health outcomes: a review. *Med Decis Making*. 2011; **31**(1): 10–8.

76. Nelson J, Cook AJ, Yu O, *et al*. Challenges in the design and analysis of sequentially-monitored post-licensure safety surveillance studies using observational health care utilization data. *Pharmacoepidemiol Drug Saf*. In press.

77. Li L, Kulldorff M, Nelson JC, Cook AJ. A propensity score-enhanced sequential analytic method for comparative drug safety surveillance. *Stat Biosci*. 2011; **3**(1): 45–62.

78. Rutter CM, Knudsen AB, Pandharipande PV. Computer disease simulation models: integrating evidence for health policy. *Acad Radiol*. 2011; **18**(9): 1077–86.

79. Carney PA, Sickles EA, Monsees BS, *et al*. Identifying minimally acceptable interpretive performance criteria for screening mammography. *Radiology*. 2010; **255**(2): 354–61.

80. White E, Miglioretti DL, Yankaskas BC, *et al*. Biennial versus annual mammography and the risk of late-stage breast cancer. *J Natl Cancer Inst*. 2004; **96**(24): 1832–9.

81. Buist DS, Anderson ML, Haneuse SJ, *et al*. Influence of annual interpretive volume on screening mammography performance in the United States. *Radiology*. 2011; **259**(1): 72–84.

82. Buist DS, Porter PL, Lehman C, *et al*. Factors contributing to mammography failure in women aged 40–49 years. *J Natl Cancer Inst*. 2004; **96**(19): 1432–40.

83. Taplin SH, Ichikawa L, Buist DS, *et al*. Evaluating organized breast cancer screening implementation: the prevention of late-stage disease? *Cancer Epidemiol Biomarkers Prev*. 2004; **13**(2): 225–34.

84. Buist DS, Anderson ML, Reed SD, *et al*. Short-term hormone therapy suspension and mammography recall: a randomized trial. *Ann Intern Med*. 2009; **150**(11): 752–65.

85. Barlow WE, White E, Ballard-Barbash R, *et al*. Prospective breast cancer risk prediction model for women undergoing screening mammography. *J Natl Cancer Inst*. 2006; **98**(17): 1204–14.

86. Wagner EH, Greene SM, Hart G, *et al*. Building a research consortium of large health systems: the Cancer Research Network. *J Natl Cancer Inst Monogr*. 2005; **35**: 3–11.

87. Wagner EH, Aiello Bowles EJ, Greene SM, *et al.* The quality of cancer patient experience: perspectives of patients, family members, providers and experts. *Qual Saf Health Care*. 2010; **19**(6): 484–9.

88. Lash TL, Fox MP, Buist DS, *et al.* Mammography surveillance and mortality in older breast cancer survivors. *J Clin Oncol.* 2007; **25**(21): 3001–6.

89. Taplin SH, Ichikawa L, Yood MU, *et al.* Reason for late-stage breast cancer: absence of screening or detection, or breakdown in follow-up? *J Natl Cancer Inst.* 2004; **96**(20): 1518–27.

90. Fenton JJ, Elmore JG, Buist DS, *et al.* Longitudinal adherence with fecal occult blood test screening in community practice. *Ann Fam Med.* 2010; **8**(5): 397–401.

91. Dublin S, Anderson ML, Haneuse SJ, *et al.* Atrial fibrillation and risk of dementia: a prospective cohort study. *J Am Geriatr Soc.* 2011; **59**(8): 1369–75.

92. Dublin S, Glazer NL, Smith NL, *et al.* Diabetes mellitus, glycemic control, and risk of atrial fibrillation. *J Gen Intern Med.* 2010; **25**(8): 853–8.

93. Lozano P, Finkelstein JA, Carey VJ, *et al.* A multisite randomized trial of the effects of physician education and organizational change in chronic-asthma care: health outcomes of the Pediatric Asthma Care Patient Outcomes Research Team II Study. *Arch Pediatr Adolesc Med.* 2004; **158**(9): 875–83.

94. Richardson LP, Russo JE, Lozano P, *et al.* Factors associated with detection and receipt of treatment for youth with depression and anxiety disorders. *Acad Pediatr.* 2010; **10**(1): 36–40.

95. Curry SJ, Ludman EJ, Graham E, *et al.* Pediatric-based smoking cessation intervention for low-income women: a randomized trial. *Arch Pediatr Adolesc Med.* 2003; **157**(3): 295–302.

96. Lieu TA, Finkelstein JA, Lozano P, *et al.* Cultural competence policies and other predictors of asthma care quality for Medicaid-insured children. *Pediatrics.* 2004; **114**(1): e102–10.

97. Glasgow RE, Orleans CT, Wagner EH. Does the chronic care model serve also as a template for improving prevention? *Milbank Q.* 2001; **79**(4): 579–612, iv–v.

98. Ralston JD, Coleman K, Reid RJ, *et al.* Patient experience should be part of meaningful-use criteria. *Health Aff (Millwood).* 2010; **29**(4): 607–13.

99. Fishman PA, Khan ZM, Thompson EE, *et al.* Health care costs among smokers, former smokers, and never smokers in an HMO. *Health Serv Res.* 2003; **38**(2): 733–49.

100. Wagner EH, Sandhu N, Newton KM, *et al.* Effect of improved glycemic control on health care costs and utilization. *JAMA.* 2001; **285**(2): 182–9.

101. Bluespruce J, Dodge WT, Grothaus L, *et al.* HIV prevention in primary care: impact of a clinical intervention. *AIDS Patient Care STDS.* 2001; **15**(5): 243–53.

102. Jackson LA, Yu O, Nelson JC, *et al.* Injection site and risk of medically attended local reactions to acellular pertussis vaccine. *Pediatrics.* 2011; **127**(3): e581–7.

103. Jackson LA, Gaglani MJ, Keyserling HL, *et al.* Safety, efficacy, and immunogenicity of an inactivated influenza vaccine in healthy adults: a randomized, placebo-controlled trial over two influenza seasons. *BMC Infect Dis.* 2010; **10**: 71.

104. Opel DJ, Taylor JA, Mangione-Smith R, *et al.* Validity and reliability of a survey to identify vaccine-hesitant parents. *Vaccine.* 2011; **29**(38): 6598–605.

105. Boudreau DM, Yu O, Johnson J. Statin use and cancer risk: a comprehensive review. *Expert Opin Drug Saf.* 2010; **9**(4): 603–21.

106. Simon GE, Ludman EJ, Tutty S, *et al.* Telephone psychotherapy and telephone care management for primary care patients starting antidepressant treatment: a randomized controlled trial. *JAMA.* 2004; **292**(8): 935–42.

107. Simon GE, Ralston JD, Savarino J, *et al.* Randomized trial of depression follow-up care by online messaging. *J Gen Intern Med.* 2011; **26**(7): 698–704.

108. Katon WJ, Lin EH, Von Korff M, *et al.* Collaborative care for patients with depression and chronic illnesses. *N Engl J Med.* 2010; **363**(27): 2611–20.

109. Arterburn DE, Westbrook EO, Bogart TA, *et al.* Randomized trial of a video-based patient decision aid for bariatric surgery. *Obesity (Silver Spring).* 2011; **19**(8): 1669–75.

110. Fishman PA, Bonomi AE, Anderson ML, *et al.* Changes in health care costs over time following the cessation of intimate partner violence. *J Gen Intern Med.* 2010; **25**(9): 920–5.

111. Grossman DC, Moyer VA, Melnyk BM, *et al.* The anatomy of a US Preventive Services Task Force Recommendation: lipid screening for children and adolescents. *Arch Pediatr Adolesc Med.* 2011; **165**(3): 205–10.

112. Riter D, Maier R, Grossman DC. Delivering preventive oral health services in pediatric primary care: a case study. *Health Aff (Millwood).* 2008; **27**(6): 1728–32.

113. Beasley JM, Ichikawa LE, Ange BA, *et al.* Is protein intake associated with bone mineral density in young women? *Am J Clin Nutr.* 2010; **91**(5): 1311–6.

114. Scholes D, LaCroix AZ, Ichikawa LE, *et al.* Injectable hormone contraception and bone density: results from a prospective study. *Epidemiology.* 2002; **13**(5): 581–7.

115. Scholes D, Grothaus L, McClure J, *et al.* A randomized trial of strategies to increase chlamydia screening in young women. *Prev Med.* 2006; **43**(4): 343–50.

5

Sparking and Sustaining the Essential Functions of Research: What Promotes Discovery?

Experience and Insights from a Medical School in China

Mengfeng Li, Guoquan Gao, Minhao Wu, Hongmei Tan, Wenjun Xin, Xia Yang, Yi Yang, Kaihua Guo, and Qiongzhu Chen*

> ### *Mengfeng Li's Story of a Success in Science: The Courage to Learn from Disagreement*
>
> About one-half year after I returned to China from the United States, where I served as a faculty member at University of Pittsburgh, my laboratory research group started here at Sun Yat-sen. I remember there was one time in the weekly lab meeting of this new group that I talked about some project ideas I wanted to pursue. Usually, we discuss the projects and the science very much in the way you would see in anyone else's university community

* **Affiliations:** From Zhongshan School of Medicine, Sun Yat-sen University, Guangzhou, Guangdong, China

Grants: This work was supported by a grant awarded to Sun Yat-sen University by the "985 Program" of Chinese Ministry of Education. The content is solely the responsibility of the authors and does not necessarily represent the official views of the Ministry of Education of China, or Sun Yat-sen University, or Zhongshan School of Medicine.

when they have lab meetings. On this particular occasion, my students (mostly PhD students or Master's students) challenged me on what I was trying to do. That challenge didn't come as a total surprise. My students and I really do sometimes disagree with each other about the science. What was striking was that they had excellent perspectives on the topic we were discussing and very good ideas. What surprised me was the *quality* of their ideas, the information they were contributing from their readings, the depth of the thinking they had been doing before that discussion, and the *new* ideas they contributed, even ideas for design of our research. Suddenly, in that moment, I realized that I actually had a really good group and that I need not worry about whether I could do research of the same or higher quality as I had been doing in Pittsburgh. That day's challenge and its follow-up brought something very significant to our science over the next 2–3 years. It turned out we produced several very good papers from this discussion, including one that I recently published in the *Journal of Clinical Investigation*. From that meeting onwards, I have tried to promote this kind of lab discussion all the time. It can happen when you host meetings and challenging discussions in small groups. I had a big laboratory group at the time, but this meeting was only of five to six people. I try to be very open to all ideas from the junior people in these small groups. Whatever they say, there are usually several important points we hear that improve our entire research activity. When I walk into that laboratory meeting room I always tell myself, "OK, now I'm one of them" – and not too far advanced to listen.

Introduction

Against a backdrop of rapid economic growth during the past three decades, scientific and technological research has gained significant momentum in China. According to the 2010 statistical data published by the People's Republic of China (PRC) Ministry of Science and Technology, between 2004 and 2009, China's research and development expenditures grew at an annual rate of 24.16% to 580.21 billion yuan; in addition, the government's science and technology appropriation increased at 24.11% per year to 322.49 billion yuan in 2009. In association with these developments, Chinese-published scientific papers cited by the Science Citation Index (SCI), Engineering Index, and Index to Scientific & Technical Proceedings indexing systems continued to skyrocket at an average yearly rate of 16.05%, 22.29% and 21.06%, respectively, to 120 000, 93 000, and 52 000 in 2009. It may be of particular note that, as is the case elsewhere in the world, biomedical science is the most dynamic and fastest growing sector in the field of science and technology in China. Such a trend is evidenced by the fact that Chinese medical and biomedical research articles indexed by MEDLINE amounted to 45 000 in 2009, up by 8.4% from 2008, and that 15.5% of these papers are labeled as "highly impacting" because they have been more frequently cited than the average publication in this sector.

For the past decade, and at a somewhat slower pace, China's major medical schools have been experiencing a transition from being teaching-oriented to research-oriented institutions. With improved scientific research facilities and conditions, new disciplinary structures, and enhanced academic development opportunities for faculty members, many of these medical schools have achieved international reputations for their scientific research. Despite these positive developments, in the view of this chapter's authors, China's scientific research system does not appear to work as efficiently as it could. For example, as the world's second largest producer of SCI-indexed papers, we believe that only a small fraction of these publications represent true scientific breakthroughs. Similarly, despite the huge number of biomedical professionals in China, only a very limited number have exerted international influence in their scientific communities.

Some of the authors of this chapter are scholars who have worked as faculty members in both US and Chinese medical schools. Because of this international experience, we have been especially interested in identifying institutional issues, solutions to which might significantly improve the cost-effectiveness of research conducted in Chinese medical schools. These issues include: (1) efficient organizational structures; (2) effective cooperation mechanisms among researchers; (3) balanced infrastructure and its full utilization; (4) a sound academic assessment system; (5) a favorable environment for development of younger scientists; and (6) a highly functional science research funding and fund-management mechanism. In this chapter we discuss organizational structure, infrastructure development, and academic assessment in the scientific research system implemented by China's medical schools, as well as their relevance to biomedical research.

Evolution of the Human Infrastructure for Scientific Research: The Principal Investigator (PI) Mechanism

For the past 50 years, exceptional changes, in breadth and depth, have taken place in the organizational structure of the scientific research system in China's medical schools.

In the 1950s a Soviet model of operating medical colleges was transferred to China's medical institutions. From the 1950s to the 1980s the Chinese version featured academic departments that were course-specific and oriented toward curriculum development and teaching. This organizational framework was adopted mainly for educational purposes, but research management was also embedded in the same system. In it all teachers in an academic department had to accept the department chairperson as both their teaching and research supervisor, for the chairperson directly led administrative operations, educational activities, and all of the few research programs that were in existence. Independent leaders of research projects were rare. In addition, scientific research funds, which were extremely limited due to an underdeveloped national economy, were allocated by the government in the form of educational funds that were committed to academic departments and therefore under the control of the department chairperson.

In the early history of the PRC this type of centralized organizational structure was important in establishing China's medical school system, and it helped the government concentrate its limited resources on urgent demands for critical science and technologies. But limited research targets and excessive bureaucratic intervention also severely undermined diversification in science, freedom, and creativity of scientific research in the 100 medical colleges and led to long-term stagnation in China's medical science research from the 1950s to the 1990s.

In 1986, when China's economic reform emerged, the National Natural Science Foundation of China (NSFC) was established, and research funds started to be directed to individuals with investigator-initiated research projects. One consequence of this shift in policy was the diversification of research project leadership, as faculty members in medical schools' academic departments were allowed to become research project leaders of their own free will, based on their scientific capabilities, not on their bureaucratic positions as medical school curriculum department heads. As time went on different international models of research management were introduced to China, and in the mid-1990s the American-style *principal investigator* mechanism made its appearance in China's medical schools. At present, this mechanism has been adopted by China's leading medical institutions as their basic organizational human infrastructure for bio-medical research. Nevertheless, it is interesting to note that the Soviet model, in various forms, still exists in many second-tier or third-tier medical colleges, largely institutions that are unable to compete successfully for external research resources. As might be expected where two different organizational models are in play, there is still controversy in the PRC about whether to continue a modi-fied former-Soviet model or to completely adopt the US PI system, although the latter has become the general trend.

In this context, it is noteworthy that, compared to the PI system in Western countries (where it first appeared), China's current PI system has its unique features. From an economic and policy standpoint, the pivotal importance of a PI system may lie in its integration in individuals of three equally important roles: achieving scientific excellence, team leadership, and institutional standing. The PI mechanism is a "three-in-one" (responsibility, capability, power) arrangement. A PI endeavors to obtain and manage resources for a project in order to ensure that its research activities are adequately funded. A PI is also the person who takes direct responsibility for completion of a funded project and must be evaluated by the institution as well as funding agencies in different ways. If academic output (for example, quality and quantity of academic publications) is not generated, the PI will be held accountable.

To ensure the fulfillment of these responsibilities, a PI should hold full power over the team in allocating resources and organizing research, such as the power to recruit, reward, punish, and dismiss his or her team members. As is the case in US medical schools, requirements for medical school PI candidates in China would ideally include competencies required to scientifically initiate and direct the research, acquire and manage financial resources for projects, and lead and manage the research team. The most important merit in this typical three-in-one mechanism is that it compels scientists to work hard for their academic goals. Despite its occasional flaws (e.g., "suppression" of the ideal to follow "free" research interest, or "ignorance" of long-term academic objectives) the PI mechanism has played an important role in facilitating the transition of some of China's top medical schools from teaching to research-oriented institutions.

Interestingly, the PI mechanism implemented in China has distinctive local features that differ from the North American version. The biggest differences may be in the preparation of the PI and how they are selected for this role. In the United States, PIs complete multi-year graduate research training experiences ("fellowships" or doctoral programs) and secure project funding by competing successfully in organized peer-review systems (e.g., at the National Institutes of

Health). While a small proportion of PIs in China's medical schools are directly recruited from biomedical institutions in Western countries, most are selected from the pool of experienced teachers or those with strong political connections and are "converted" into PIs. As many of the "old-style" faculty members may not be completely capable of succeeding in the three required abilities (academic, resource-acquisition, and organizing abilities), some schools opt for stability at the expense of competency. As a result the definition and appointment of PIs in China's medical schools are usually subject to non-academic and non-competency factors like seniority, popularity, social/community connections, and political power that may result in the unjust acquisition of resources.

Another flaw in China's new PI mechanism is the lack of integration of PIs' responsibility, function, and power in a three-in-one arrangement. Under its current personnel management system and research-funding policy, PIs have only very limited power in hiring team associates and assistants or deciding their salaries. This is partly due to the low proportion of China's research funding allocated to human resources and the heavy dependency on recruitment of team members with limited administrative resources. As a result, research teams usually consist of up to 90% less experienced graduate students and few, if any, experienced post-docs or research associates. These conditions often result in research underperformance and – at the same time – the expanding enrollments and demand for more teaching has produced high student-to-teacher ratios in China's medical schools, a discouraging situation, at best, for PIs who have their sights set on research careers.

Whatever its limitations, the Chinese version of the PI system is still functioning as an important catalyst in advancing China's biomedical research. One specific example can be seen at Sun Yat-sen University (SYSU), where a PI-based research system in health science schools was implemented in 2003. The number of SCI-indexed articles published by SYSU biomedical and clinical scientists has doubled in three years. A hoped-for and important effect of the PI system at SYSU, and elsewhere in China, is that competition has become the major driving force for scientific innovation. A second "by-product" of the adoption of this system is that it has contributed to attracting Chinese-born biomedical scientists who work and study abroad (such as the authors!) to return home to establish their research teams and careers as PIs in China's medical schools.

Prior to the PI system implementation the annual productivity at SYSU in terms of publications in international journals was fewer than 200 per year. Since 2003, when the PI mechanism was first applied to its research management system, its SCI-cited papers and funded projects have been multiplying annually, exceeding 1000 in 2009. Some of these publications have appeared in world-recognized academic journals such as the *New England Journal of Medicine*, *Science*, *Nature Genetics*, *Nature Biotechnology*, *Journal of Clinical Investigation*, *PNAS*, *Lancet*, *Cell*, *Blood*, and *Circulation Research*.

The gradual transition from the previous teaching-oriented departmental structure to a research-oriented PI-based operational system represents a fundamental shift in the management approach of China's medical schools. While Chinese biomedical research has benefited from the implementation of the new PI mechanism, the system, as it is currently manifested in China's medical schools, is still in its infancy, works sub-optimally and faces many challenges.

- The current "transition" from the Soviet to the PI system in China allows the appointment of "sub-competent" PIs, resulting in inappropriate resource allocation, poor academic output, and little scientific innovation.

- A special challenge for the current PI system is finding ways to build and enhance clinical scientist-led research teams. Most medical school physicians are insufficiently trained in research methods and are therefore "unqualified" to be PIs. Were qualified clinician-scientists available they could identify meaningful medical and health questions amenable to basic, translational, and clinical research. This problem, together with the inadequate research infrastructure and resources allocated to and "owned" by clinical departments, represents a major difficulty in implementing effective translational research programs.

- The PI system at present also suffers from limitations in the composition of individual PI teams. Under the current system the majority of team members are postgraduate students (usually at the master's level), themselves in need of training, but who staff the middle layer in the ecological system of a PI team, while skilled postdoctoral researchers are rare. This state of affairs is related to the lack of support from the funding system as the majority of domestic research funds exclude salaries for junior scientists.

- An additional PI system challenge is that under the current research-based assessment system, mandated in China's higher education institutions, PIs, especially junior PIs, are incentivized to maximize early publication at the cost of their true interests in science and invest only limited, if any, effort in those fundamentally important issues which might take a long time to generate significant results.

- Finally, team spirit, one of the keys to scientific breakthroughs, has yet to be encouraged and protected. Built upon the current accountability system, the PI mechanism utilizes competition as a major driving force in the pursuit of higher academic performance. Overemphasizing the usefulness of competition may easily harm scientific research as a whole, as has been the case in many other countries, including the United States. It is imperative that attention and effort be invested in devising effective ways to motivate the PIs to work more closely with one another for a broader academic vision and substantial scientific breakthroughs.

In summary, in spite of its strengths and important contributions, it is clear that measures must be taken to improve the current PI-based operational system in Chinese medical schools. Most importantly, selection and appointment of PIs prepared and qualified for their "three-in-one" responsibilities must be solidly enforced and founded upon internationally recognized criteria. To that end, an effective peer-review mechanism must be implemented, perhaps by integrating international peer reviewers, to provide fair and equitable methods for making merit-based decisions about distributing resources. In addition, governmental regulation and policies for using research funds should be reformed to ensure that PIs have the final say on the employment and periodic evaluation of research team members.

Importantly, academic cooperation should be incorporated into the assessment of PIs to facilitate collaborations among PIs, particularly interdisciplinary collaborations. It is also particularly important for China's medical schools, like their international counterparts, to address the challenge in building an effective framework for institutionalizing ways to narrow the huge divide between basic science PIs and clinicians as two different interest groups. Some Chinese medical schools have taken on this challenge and have created disease-oriented research units which accommodate basic science PIs, physician scientists, clinical researchers, and translational technologists under one umbrella. These units may be important "incubators" for the next generation of PI-led research efforts in the evolution of Chinese medical school research.

The Impact of an Index-based Evaluation System and Incentives for Scientific Discovery in China's Medical Schools

Institutional policies and culture are always needed to ensure that scientists are appropriately evaluated and adequately incentivized in their pursuit of academic achievement. The incentive mechanism for scientific research in China has gone through three stages since the 1950s.

A Government-led Incentive Mechanism before the 1980s

From 1940 to the 1980s, a highly centralized, government-oriented incentive mechanism was established in scientific research under a centrally planned national economy. The basic rationale for this type of incentive mechanism was the principle of "gathering strength to make major breakthroughs." In a society where political belief was supreme, only very few scientists, recognized as politically trustworthy, would have the opportunity to be provided with some political, ideological, and economic incentives. Under such an evaluation and incentive mechanism, chances for success were only given to those who were: (1) "science fanatics" who did not need incentives anyway; (2) political idealists or patriots who also had a certain degree of interest in science; (3) political specu-lators (those who intend to "profit" politically by their actions) in the academic community; and (4) people with any combination of the three characteristics. Unfortunately, such an incentive mechanism did nothing to incentivize passion and innovation for science, a particularly serious challenge for Chinese society, a country with 20% of the world's population.

Early Stage Performance-based Assessment System (the end of the 1970s to the early 2000s)

About the same time that China's economic reform began in the 1980s, incen-tives for scientific research in academic settings started to be reformed. The traditional politics-centered, government-led incentive mechanism was gradually replaced by a performance-based assessment system through decentralization of power and resources. Due to underdeveloped academic institutions, a struggling national economy, and stagnant international academic cooperation, academic success was mostly domestic and the performance assessment system was focused primarily around publications in Chinese-language journals. Despite the absence of an international peer-review process, the academic value of the papers published during this period was still somewhat quality-controlled, and journals had to pay authors to publish their articles. The number of domestically circulating journals was small, with only approximately 100 biomedical and medi-cal journals registered as "Core Journals" in the *Chinese Science and Technology Data Directory – Medical and Health Volume* in 1978. At the same time, library access for Chinese scientists to international journals remained limited due to their high cost.

This situation prevailed until the mid-1990s when widespread changes in incentives led to a plethora of new domestic journals (skyrocketing to over 600, not including the large number of local journals and published conference proceedings). In addition, during this period journals began to profit from page charges. These factors, together with many others, had a profound negative effect on the domestic peer-review system and Chinese biomedical/medical journals rapidly lost their academic quality and reputation.

Dawn of the 21st Century, and an Index-based Evaluation and Incentive Mechanism

With a rising investment in research in a rapidly growing economy, scientific discoveries made in China began to be recognized in the international arena, as evidenced by the growing number of peer-reviewed papers authored by Chinese scientists and indexed by internationally recognized databases, such as the Science Citation Index. A parallel international index-based incentive/appraisal mechanism has appeared in China and it has established a leading presence in its major higher education institutions and research institutes. These trends have been effective in preventing further deterioration in the value of scientific papers published in domestic journals. At the same time, international recognition of Chinese research seems to have had impact on biomedical research that is positive and multidimensional. Biomedical scientists are encouraged or even "forced" to publish in high impact-factor journals regardless of the academic fields they are in. Many medical colleges in China give their faculty members extra monetary incentives if their papers are indexed by SCI. For example, since 2002, a leading medical college in China has been rewarding its faculty members with cash of different amounts based on the SCI impact factor of the journal in which a paper is published, with a 10 000 RMB (yuan) incentive per one impact factor point. Interestingly, in a few medical colleges' evaluation of academic papers faculty members are required to be accurate to several decimal places, leading some in China's scientific community to call the SCI the "Stupid Chinese Index."

Quantitative indices, represented by the SCI impact factor, have been extensively used in annual and service-term evaluations as well as in the promotion assessment of medical school teachers. For example, in quite a few medical schools, to pass service-term assessments and obtain a contract renewal, faculty members are required to have publications in journals with a certain impact factor (≥ 3–5, for example). Faculty members who fail in the assessment may have their allowances cut, or be transferred or dismissed by these colleges. Interestingly, the SCI impact factor also plays a decisive role in the recruitment of new faculty members. It is not uncommon for some post-doctoral fellows or newly graduated doctoral students, who have not demonstrated an independently strong academic capability, to be employed as full professors, only because they worked in internationally leading laboratories and published papers in high-impact-factor journals. The significance of SCI publications and the related journal impact factors have been strongly and directly felt in almost all academic awards at the institutional level and the national level. The SCI-based incentive mechanism seems to have been implemented everywhere.

The SCI-based mechanism became so widely accepted in China in the context of an academic environment in which huge amounts of research were published in domestic journals without fair and critical peer review. In an academic community without an international peer-review system, an immature domestic peer-review culture, and defective peer-review rules, adoption of an easily implemented assessment system based on quantitative and comparable metrics readily lowered political costs and avoided direct institutional responsibility. The SCI-based mechanism was an easy choice for most institutions.

The SCI is accepted in China as an objective assessment standard. Depending on their highly professional and impartial editors, strict editing and publishing rules, and independent international peer review, leading international journals endeavor to ensure that only innovative papers with a sophisticated design, a reliable methodology and credible results are published. An academic paper that is published in a high-impact-factor journal and cited frequently by international colleagues is recognized as credible and significant in the international arena. Despite the fact that the impact factor of a journal cannot be directly used to measure the impact of individual articles it publishes, the indexing approach with accurate numeric metrics remains attractive to the medical colleges where quantitative standards are needed to assess researchers.

Has the SCI-based incentive mechanism been a catalyst for science research in China's medical colleges? Despite the drawbacks of using an exclusively SCI-based approach to assess productivity in Chinese medical schools, this practice has contributed to the advancement of biomedical research in China. For example, in their effort to publish in fine journals, the professional vision and capabilities of researchers, some of whom had been inadequately trained to conduct independent research, can improve, along with their writing and communication skills. These same faculty members are incentivized to engage more actively in scientific discovery. Since a SCI-based assessment and incentive system was initiated by SYSU health science schools and hospitals in 2003 the number of SCI-indexed papers has increased steadily to nearly 1000 in 2010. Along with publication have come increased academic influence and more competitive funding awards. Our research programs and their academic value are increasingly acknowledged by the international community.

What are some of the limitations of an index-based incentive mechanism? One important demonstration of the true value of a scientific discovery is the social and economic benefits it brings. In this sense, an index-based assessment and incentive mechanism has limitations, because impact factors only reflect the innovation and value of a scientific discovery in indirect ways. Excessive use of index-based evaluation standards may also constrain the fulfillment of long-term research targets. The "all for SCI" attitude may bend scientific research to the sole purpose of publication and lure researchers to turn to some "hot" topics with shorter research time horizons, easier procedures, and quicker returns while staying away from those requiring a long time to bear fruit.

Overemphasis on SCI impact factor may also impede applied research that often requires large investments of manpower, resources, and money over a longer period of time to produce results. Such research does not often demonstrate its value and benefits in academic articles in short order. As a case in point, the discovery of artemisinin, an anti-malaria drug, was the result of tremendous investment over a long period of time. Through the 1960s and 70s numerous researchers devoted their energy to the search for such a medicine. They consulted countless medical books of all ages and veteran doctors and tried thousands of traditional Chinese regimens before identifying the artemisinin compound in the herb *Artemisia annua*. The chemical was finally isolated after more than 190 attempts. The drug developed is the most effective anti-malarial available today. Without generating any high-impact SCI papers it has saved millions of lives worldwide, especially in developing countries, and eventually won the Lasker Medical Research Award.

It is also true that inappropriate use of an index-based evaluation system may in many ways reshape the intentions and perspectives of researchers in scientific collaboration. The current motivating mechanism in China tends to use a simple quantitative standard to determine accurately the share of contribution of each person on a research team. Beneficiaries of the index-based incentive mechanism are mainly corresponding authors and first authors. Disputes over this issue are not uncommon, and such non-academic considerations can lead to abortion of valuable large-scale major projects that require close cooperation among multiple academic disciplines and research teams.

In summary, while an index-based quantitative academic incentive and assessment mechanism, which precludes political intervention and potentially unfair distribution of resources, represents a relatively fair, objective, and internationally accepted arrangement, it does not do so without creating its own potentially significant challenges. How the dilemma and contradiction can be effectively handled, or balanced, has become an issue faced by all medical school deans and academic administrations in China.

The Special Importance of Optimally Established Research Facilities in China's Medical Schools

There is no doubt that contemporary biomedicine is increasingly dependent on the excellence of its research infrastructure, including research equipment and service facilities. Research infrastructure per se has become an important indication in the evaluation of a medical school or college and the accreditation of its medical education. In China, the scientific research infrastructure is particularly important because the nation is working hard to achieve its biomedical ambitions and, in some circumstances, still coping with the residual effects of a less developed economy.

Since the 1950s, bricks and mortar construction for scientific research in China's medical schools has gone through three phases of development. The first one lasted from the 1950s till the 1980s. In the first phase, the general level of research infrastructure was at least 20 years behind that in the developed countries, largely due to the limited investment of financial resources in scientific research, an extremely underdeveloped national economy, and the lack of advanced technologies and equipment due to China's political and economic isolation from the developed world.

Since the 1980s, China has initiated economic reforms and opened its market to the outside world, in the hope of catching up. Advanced research technologies and equipment were introduced to China, along with rapidly increasing international exchanges, in almost all business areas. As a result the world's leading manufacturers of research equipment began to establish markets in China. During this period, a number of medical colleges and research institutes in China were outfitted with imported research equipment, and a handful of institutions even purchased high-end biomedical research devices.

Today the scientific research infrastructure in most major medical colleges has been upgraded to international standards, thanks to the tremendous investment made through such government initiatives as Program 985 and Program 211. Since 2000, China's expenditure in science research and experimental development has risen by 23% per year to 580.21 billion yuan in 2009. A huge investment has been made by China's universities both in purchasing advanced equipment and in the autonomous development of research equipment. The total value of science research equipment owned by China's universities in 2005 was 5.4 times higher than that in 1995. All major manufacturers of scientific instruments now view China as one of their most important markets.

With research infrastructure development accelerated in China's medical schools, problems and misconceptions are also emerging behind the splendid hardware upgrades. For example, there is a lack of appropriate assessment of where and how to invest, which often leads to redundant and low-level construction. Moreover, the absence of an infrastructure sharing mechanism, the lack of a culture of sharing, and an imbalance between development and maintenance budgets, has led to low efficiency, which is represented by a generally low average usage time and limited researcher access to facilities. These problems not only can directly impede the output and efficiency of biomedical research, they also may undermine the enthusiasm of faculty members in pursuing research in indirect ways, as they lead to perceptions of unfairness sensed among faculty members and students.

It is also worth noting that China's current investment in scientific resources has entered a "developed" stage, an ironic circumstance for a country whose economy is still considered as "developing" in most areas. It is understood that the country has limited available resources compared to the developed countries; however, this contrasts sharply with the country's great ambition for hardware construction to improve science and technology and stimulate academic output. Hopefully, this conundrum will motivate leaders and administrators of Chinese medical schools to work together and explore and design more effective solutions for resource management and, where possible, resource-sharing. This kind of sharing, however, will not be easy, and reports of success are important to highlight.

The challenge of enhancing efficient use of research facilities in China's medical schools goes far beyond resource-constraint problems such as inappropriate budget allocation and limited space availability; it also relates to deeper problems rooted in the academic culture of the scientific community and the operational systems of medical schools, which also involve the incentive/performance assessment mechanisms. In 2008, SYSU Zhongshan School of Medicine began to develop a system named *Automated Comprehensive Common Equipment Sharing System* (ACCESS) to facilitate facility-sharing. By integrating user authorization, reservation management, instrument operation, technical training, and billing services into a highly automatic platform, ACCESS has networked nearly 200 research instruments and core facilities (such as animal facility, high-grade biosafety facility, and radioactive manipulation laboratory) that are completely open to all researchers and research assistants. When a device is switched on by a user card, the system automatically records the user's information, the device in use, and technical status of the device. Meanwhile, the PC interface of ACCESS enables each instrument to publish its basic technical parameters, physical location, and current and future reservations to hundreds of PI and thousands of users through the network, accept reservations 24/7 in a fully open fashion without administrative intervention, and also provides a real-time billing service for each device in a real-time manner. In addition, through the ACCESS host computer at the Command Center, the system administrator is able to acquire information on operation of all the devices, and with the help of the automatically captured information on the use of the devices, the school is also able to identify the most needed devices and make purchase decisions based on an evidence-based assessment. At the same time, through the PI terminal, the PIs are able to acquire information regarding how the devices are used by their associates and students. Such information seems quite useful for PIs to improve their lab management and project progress. Experience gained from operating the ACCESS network platform suggests that certain "rules" might be important and generalizable when attempting to implement an effective facility-sharing system in China's medical schools.

- Rule No 1: All administrative and user roles should be clearly separated to ensure that all users are equal. PIs, as well as their associates, should not be included in the administrative part of the system. In fact, at SYSU medical school's current ACCESS system, it takes only four carefully selected, school-paid technicians to fulfill all the management tasks for the entire system.
- Rule No. 2: All charges and fees paid by PIs should not go directly to the ACCESS office. The ACCESS is built and maintained purely through the school's budget, and the income collected through the use of ACCESS should never be used as a performance parameter when evaluating the operation of the system. The revenue generated from the use of devices should properly go to the general school account and is not connected to the income of ACCESS staff. It is interesting to note that although only a significant fee is charged for each use of each device we have never received any complaints about our rates. It is well-known that the collection of these fees contributes significantly to the school budget, and in a purely numeric sense, they are completely able to cover the maintenance of the system.
- Rule No. 3: Technology is important for the successful and sustainable maintenance of a sharing system. Appropriate sharing technology plays a key role in the automation of the entire system, which is crucial in making the system

open, fair, efficient, and transparent, particularly in China's academic cultural environment.

Since it was put into operation in 2009, ACCESS has hosted an average of 10 000 users and logged about 40 000 machine hours of use per year. Currently, common and less expensive devices (e.g., centrifuges, real-time PCR machines, microplate readers), mid-level equipment (e.g., flow-cytometric analyzer, the Luminex), and high-end instruments (e.g., laser-captured micro-dissection sets, confocal microscopes, patch clamps), are all shared on an automated basis under ACCESS. The system is being further optimized and expanded to ensure higher levels of efficiency and cost-effectiveness.

Summary

The environments of academic organizations motivate scientists and promote scientific discovery. These human, policy, and physical environments are critical to discovery and application of findings from research. Our own experience in leading and managing a major medical school with the longest medical education history in China has been interesting, particularly when comparing the macro-environment in which it is currently run with those in North America and other developed countries.

China continues to experience revolutionary changes in many aspects. One such change dynamic is the rapid development and further opening up of Chinese society and its economy, a process that is bringing dramatic changes to how resources are distributed and managed in academic institutions and health science centers. Against a background of rapid advances in biomedicine there are increasing demands for better health among China's citizens. If they are to suc-ceed in responding to this demand in a timely way, China's medical schools will need to upgrade everything that is critical to their scientific programs, including organizational structure, researcher assessment, and management skills.

In this chapter we have discussed some of the intra-institutional improve-ments that have been instituted from the perspective of one of China's leading medical schools. These reforms have helped mend some innate flaws inherited from the previous operating model and open the school to international medical education and academic communities. We would caution that the implemen-tation of such measures is always subject to the fundamental restrictions of macro-environmental factors, such as science policies, health policies, and human resource management policies, which make reforms at the national and governmental levels essential.

It must be noted that some problems in the administration of a medical school, such as the institutional barriers that contribute to the lack of interdisciplinary cooperation and slow translational research, exist not only in China but also in many other countries. They are the "Deans' headaches" in almost all health science centers and medical schools worldwide. To overcome these barriers, medical colleges from different political systems and cultural backgrounds will need to work more closely and learn more from each other so as to achieve the goal of promoting discoveries key to the enhancement of human health and well-being.

Acknowledgment

We thank Drs. Richard Frankel and Thomas Inui for their significant and important editing work on this chapter.

References

- Institute of Scientific and Technical Information of China, Statistical Data of Chinese S&T Papers. Available at: www.sts.org.cn/sjkl/kjtjdt/
- Ministry of Science and Technology of the People's Republic of China, China Science & Technology Statistics. Available at: www.sts.org.cn/sjkl/kjtjdt/index.htm

6

Sparking and Sustaining the Essential Functions of Research

How the Seeds were Sown and Grown at a Summer Camp for Young Clinicians

Shunichi Fukuhara

Shunichi Fukuhara's Story of a Success in Science: Following Your Dreams

Ten years after I graduated from medical school I took the Clinical Effectiveness summer curriculum, a joint program of Harvard Medical School and the Harvard School of Public Health. I continued in my studies there and received the MPH degree. This was very valuable experience for me because it changed my career. Before then, I had been a 100% clinician, but that program put me on a clinician-investigator path. After that experience I thought of myself as a clinical epidemiologist and a health-services researcher, both of which are definitely lacking in Japan. I realized that nobody learns this kind of science in medical school in Japan, and I felt that some day it should be introduced into Japanese medical education and/or postgraduate training. I never dreamt that I would be the pioneer for that introduction, except maybe somewhere in my subconscious.

Over time I began to feel that this innovation in education was certainly necessary. When I was at the University of Tokyo, with my educator colleague Joe Green I offered a seminar course to teach clinical research design to master's and PhD students in the graduate school of medicine. It was 1996.

> That offering attracted almost no attention. Most of the students were from foreign countries. This was very disappointing, but still I felt strongly that this type of teaching program was going to be necessary. I remember outlining my dreams on a whiteboard to review with Joe Green. Even now we reminisce about that day. I told Joe that in Japan we needed some academic center for health research, not just biological research. He and I were laughing because it seemed a ridiculous idea when we had just given a seminar to which almost no Japanese students came. He suggested that the idea and vision were correct, but that the time and place might not be right. Not too long afterward, I accepted an appointment and department chair's position at Kyoto University. From that point on, the story again had ups and downs, and is described in the chapter I have written for this book.

The Context (a Very Brief History)

This is a small story that takes place in a country far from Western civilization, a country that closed itself off from the rest of the world from the 1600s until the end of the 1800s – almost 300 years. While this country was closed, medical care was provided mainly by herb prescribers, who were the ancestors of physicians in Japan.

At the end of the 1800s Japan began looking to the West for new ideas in science, medicine, and emerging technologies. The government at that time looked at medical care and medical education in several European countries and decided to import a particular German style of academic medicine. There were really only two imports the government considered: particular values and a particular structure. In terms of values, they imported what was a kind of "biomedical absolutism," by which I mean prioritizing the discovery of a single, objective, fundamental cause of a disease, and ultimately finding a cure. In terms of structure, it imported a top-down, academy-centric style. The latter defined the social responsibility of academic medicine. The mission of the Imperial University of Tokyo, for example, was to create professors for other new universities. Its mission was to disseminate the 19th-century values of Western medicine from the top down, throughout Japan.

Were those two imports accurate and complete representations of German academic medicine, or did they reflect an official, skewed, and truncated view that satisfied the preferences of Japan's government at that time? That is a question I leave to professional historians. In either case, these two imports had profound effects on Japanese medicine. First, academic medicine in Japan was established as a laboratory-centered practice, which influenced the kinds of knowledge it fostered. For example, laboratory parasitology leads directly to knowledge about parasites in a laboratory. From it, one learns nothing (directly) about the risks of disease or its effects on clinical populations. Second, academic medicine in Japan was established as hierarchical in at least two ways: the top-down relation of the main national universities to other universities, and the top-down human relations within departments – each with a single professor at the top of a pyramid of social status. Having been imported from the West, both biomedical absolutism and the top-down structure among and within universities could easily be justified as "modernization."

More than a century and two world wars have passed since Japan became "modernized," and we can appropriately ask, what medical values should Japan embrace? Of course we still value science, but in my view we should place more emphasis on what I call "probabilism." Even laboratory science has moved away from simple cause-effect models. Instead of discovering a single cause of a disease, we now try to estimate the importance of various risk factors and the likelihoods of various effects of treatments in a complex web of phenomena. Instead of thinking that we can conquer a disease, we do what we can to reduce its incidence and prevalence, to manage its symptoms, and to lessen the burden it imposes on individuals and society. In terms of structures, in this century we now look to the "grass roots," trying to identify unmet needs in communities. We also value human resources from the bottom up; that is, local health-care providers such as physicians serving in their communities. In contemporary academic health-science centers, our responsibility is to teach the skills of critical and analytical thinking and to empower our students to do research based on their own practice or on community health-care policy. We should make every effort to return these human resources and the fruit of their work back to their communities.

Something New at Kyoto University

Those observations of the past and the present were in my head when I started working at Kyoto University in the year 2000. The university was founded in 1897, as Japan's second Imperial University. To date, it has placed a very strong emphasis on laboratory science (even stronger than the University of Tokyo), in some sense preserving the 19th-century value of "biomedical absolutism." The emphasis on laboratory research continued even after World War II, when the strongest influences began to come not from Europe but from America. The results have been good, at least by the standards of laboratory science. For example, Professor Susumu Tonegawa of Kyoto University is an eminent immunologist and a Nobel-prize laureate, and Professor Shinya Yamanaka led the team that generated the first induced pluripotent stem cells. In doing so, they may have established an entirely new form of treatment in modern medicine.

In 2000 a School of Public Health was founded at Kyoto University. Given the 19th-century values and structure that predominated at that time, the School of Public Health was really a misfit. It was another step away from absolutism and toward probabilism, from laboratory experiments to community issues. I moved to this School of Public Health, and five years later we took the second step. Our group started the Master's Program in Clinical Research (MCR) inside that School. This also had never been done before, and it was a further misfit both in the university as a whole and also in the School of Public Health. We called it "Misfit squared" (Misfit^2).

My colleagues and I started the MCR program from zero. We had no seed money, no new faculty, no new staff, no reputation, and no precedent. But we did have confidence in our mission, which is based on 21st-century values and structure, and we also had a few like-minded friends in the School of Public Health. We were sure that there were latent needs in communities throughout Japan. We knew that starting this new program would be risky (the Dean said: "Succeed or perish"), but in 2005 we took the risk. We started the MCR program as an experiment. What happened? From inside Kyoto University we were completely ignored. From outside, we got 15 applicants for five student openings and by the end of the first five years of the program we had graduated 60 students, all of them clinicians.

Some outcomes of the program have certainly been good. For example, MCR program alumni have written at least 80 research articles that were published in international, peer-reviewed journals. Also, more than half of the alumni are now in PhD programs or have already become medical school faculty themselves. One has even become a full professor. We were pleased to see that almost 40% of our graduates went back to their home towns, to work in community hospitals and clinics. However, in a 2008 alumni survey we discovered that there was still a gap between what we were teaching and our graduates' skills and abilities to do research in their communities. Specifically, our alumni indicated that they do not have enough time to do research and that they are not appreciated as researchers. In fact, some of their colleagues believe that any work other than clinical work is worthless. In essence, this group has no infrastructure to support clinical research, no support for data analysis or for writing, and, of course, they have no money. In fact, people say to them, "Why do you need money to do clinical research? You should be able to do it without any funding." Clearly, our achievements were less than completely satisfactory. In "Sustaining Change" (p. 105), I will describe how we are dealing with these new challenges.

In Japan, the Ministry of Education controls the number of students that an academic program can accept. When it began, the MCR program did not have any new slots for students. For the first few years, all of the MCR students were admitted into slots that had been assigned to the more general master's program in the School of Public Health. In 2008, the MCR program was approved by the Ministry of Education, which created a few slots explicitly and exclusively for students to be admitted to the MCR program. From 2008 to 2010, two more departments joined the MCR program. Connections also began to develop between the MCR program and another program, one with no formal relation to Kyoto University. We called it the "summer camp."

Summer Camp, Part 1

The opportunity that triggered the creation of the summer camp came unexpectedly. I happened to have been involved, as a member of the steering committee, in a large research project on end-stage renal disease, called the Dialysis Outcomes and Practice Patterns Study (DOPPS). This project was funded by a non-profit foundation in Japan. One day I was in a foundation board meeting that had been called to discuss issues regarding promoting outcomes research in Japan, particularly in renal diseases, separately from the DOPPS study. The board members discussed how this foundation could use its funds most effectively, and one board member asked whether and how this foundation was contributing to young people's education or training in outcomes research. It was not on the agenda, but five or six minutes were spent discussing this issue.

I hadn't prepared to discuss this issue at all, but for years I had been longing for an opportunity to start a program to educate young clinicians in the theory and skills of clinical research. I really didn't care which fields or sub-specialty it began in (nephrology, cardiology, primary care, etc.), I just wanted to start that kind of a program. So I raised my hand and proposed a rough idea that the foundation might support an educational program outside academia to teach young nephrologists something about outcomes research during the summer. I was the youngest board member and I am not a nephrologist, so I didn't expect the older board members, all of whom were real authorities in that field, to support this idea. But, again unexpectedly, they supported it and they asked me to make a more substantial proposal.

More Recent Background

As described above, medical education in Japan has not emphasized probabilistic reasoning or the application of epidemiological and statistical thinking in clinical practice. This could be one reason why Japan has been very weak when it comes to clinical research. Recently, that weakness seems to have gotten worse. For example, the number of original articles from Japan that were published in 120 "clinical core journals" has declined over the past five years, while it has been rising for China and Korea. How did physicians in Japan ever learn anything about how to do clinical research? A few went abroad, and a few of those who went abroad (very few, actually) studied clinical epidemiology and clinical research rather than laboratory methods, but they were very much the exceptions.

For the most part, virtually all that Japanese physicians learned about clinical research came from textbooks. Of course, no complex skill can be easily learned from a textbook alone. Those in Tokyo might have been able to attend one-day or two-day events featuring eminent foreign academics. These events were often called "seminars," but in fact they were didactic unidirectional (top-down) lectures given in English with some explanations in Japanese. I had attended several of these events, and I strongly suspected that most of the attendees (I can't really call them "participants") did not understand the content of the lectures and were not completely satisfied with the form of the event. Recognizing that this type of approach was doomed to fail, I wanted to create a type of program that had never before existed in Japan.

I decided to produce a program organized as follows:

1. Participants should have at least five years' clinical training and should be younger than age 40. The reason was that I wanted to recruit people who had enough experience to know what is and isn't clinically important but who were not so senior that they would be looking forward to retirement.

2. The summer camp should last at least 5, and ideally 7 days. It should be a residential program, off campus, and participants should have official written approval from their director or professor to be completely free from all clinical duties during that time.

3. This summer camp should have 8 participants (a maximum of 12). In order to cast as wide a net as possible, applications should be welcomed from all over Japan. Announcements should be made available through the Internet, in journals, and in other media of academic associations and clinical societies.

4. It is important that all education be provided in the Japanese language. There were many reasons for this decision. Using Japanese frees participants from dependence on translation and interpretation. I thought that they would also be more at ease asking questions and having conversation during "off" hours. Using Japanese also leads to greater sustainability since faculty members are available for long-term follow-up. There is also less chance for intimidation (conscious or not) by teachers who are assumed to be infallible experts.

5. Participants should not call each other "Dr. XXX." Instead they should choose a nickname, which is something that they would never do on their own. The participants should come from different institutions and different geographic areas. The goal was to erase part of the old identity and put things on a more casual footing. This also includes not allowing institutional or geographic cliques to form and reinforce one another. This might be particularly important in Japan, because this country is highly centralized and focused on the Tokyo area. I wanted to make sure we did not sharpen that focus, because the periphery is at least as valuable as the center.

6. In principle, faculty members and education facilitators should stay together with the participants and stay throughout the program, to reinforce the idea that we were creating a community. Everyone needs to keep their attention on the summer camp alone.

7. Participants, faculty members, and facilitators should sign a document pledging that they will not utilize this community for any "political" purpose. That means it should not be used to make a voting bloc in academic societies and the like. I thought this was important because creating a new community is easier if we start from zero, and this particular community should emphasize academic content and commonality of clinical interest over any power-based affiliation.

8. This program should have no direct connection with any university. Instead, it was supported and organized by a non-profit organization, the Institute for Health Outcomes and Process Evaluation research (iHope international). That organization receives its funds from the outcomes-research foundation and it is obliged to report its activities and outcomes. I founded iHope in 2004. Its objectives are very similar to the missions and goals of my department at Kyoto University. I founded iHope because there are many

administrative and legal barriers that prohibit national universities from doing innovative outreach activities using their own mechanisms of financial support. A new law regarding non-profit organizations had recently taken effect, so the timing was good and the government encouraged these organizations to do activities that had not been possible inside existing educational and research institutes under the old law. Specifically, it would not have been possible for the summer camp to be an activity of the university, but iHope could do it. For reasons of transparency, and to prevent conflicts of interest between sponsor and learners, the summer-camp program has an advisory committee made up of board members of the outcomes-research foundation.

Goals of the Summer Camp

There were two long-term goals, as follows.
1. To create a new community of young clinical researchers in Japan.
2. To communicate a substantial quantity of high-quality, clinically relevant, research results from Japan to the world.

There were four short-term goals for after the summer camp.
1. More than half of the participants would continue to communicate with each other, maintaining networks.
2. About 10%–20% of the participants would decide to continue their learning systematically by enrolling in graduate schools or taking part in distance-learning programs.
3. Among those who would continue their study, some would start their own research projects.
4. Some of the research projects would yield published results in top-tier journals.

To achieve those short-term goals, I did three things. First, I established a website and a mailing list for summer-camp alumni. Second, I started holding an alumni forum at the time of the annual meeting of the Nephrology Society where past attendees could report on their activities over the past year. This also included a poster competition of the abstracts presented at the meeting and an award for the best abstract. I also invited outside clinicians or researchers to attend plenary talks given by past attendees. Third, I produced and published an annual report of the summer camp. The report has follow-up information on alumni, including abstracts and original articles produced each year, and a summary of the latest summer camp.

Learning Objectives and Curriculum

The summer camp had five learning objectives.
1. To understand the essentials of clinical research. For example, it was necessary to dispel the misunderstandings that clinical research must involve a randomized controlled trial and that learning biostatistical skills is enough to resolve most problems in clinical research.
2. To learn the basic elements of epidemiology and biostatistics as they are applied in clinical research.
3. To recognize that the most important part of the whole process of clinical research is not computing the right statistics, but designing and constructing a good conceptual framework or "blueprint" for the research.
4. By the end of the summer camp, each participant should have completed a research plan for a project.
5. To know when and how to consult with specialists (such as a biostatistician).

With these learning goals in mind, we constructed a 1-week curriculum. It consisted mainly of didactic lectures and practical training in principles and practices of clinical research. It included epidemiology, biostatistics, and research ethics; in addition, we put a lot of emphasis on how to translate a vague clinical question into a research question that can be answered.

Life in Summer Camp

Students spent all day in classes and in practical training. All participants had breakfast, lunch, and dinner together with the faculty and staff. During the evenings they prepared for the final day, when they had to present their research plan. The students worked very hard and the faculty and staff supported them. Students were given one half day off completely, when they were allowed to leave the facility. Some of them played golf together and some groups went for a walk and a chat. At first, they were afraid to communicate openly because they came from entirely different areas and institutions. But, as time went by, they became friendly and by the end they had become very close.

On the final day, very famous professors came to the camp to judge the presentations, and the students were very anxious. When the presentations were over, the one or two best speakers were selected by the judges. Then we had a "graduation" ceremony and a party. It was a moving moment, which was much more emotional than we expected it to be, and some of the students even cried.

Short-term Outcomes

After the summer camp, the participants returned to their home institutions excited and highly motivated. The mailing list communication was active. We also got some very positive feedback from directors of their institutions: "His attitude changed. His eyes shone and his interest in clinical work improved remarkably." This type of remark was unexpected because the aim of this summer camp was to promote clinical research. But we were pleasantly surprised to find that it influenced participants' attitude and behavior in clinical practice too.

The initial excitement did not last long. There was a honeymoon period of only 1–2 months, and then most participants began to be preoccupied with their regular daily clinical work, and mailing list communication rapidly decreased. All of us on the faculty and staff were extremely interested to know whether the alumni continued their study or research. We even organized a small follow-up meeting 4–5 months after the summer camp, and found out that most of the students did not continue their study or research work. This was disappointing.

Still, there were some successes. One of the summer camp students contacted me and said that he had decided to come to Kyoto University to learn clinical research systematically, starting with the MCR program and moving on to the PhD program. In Japan, it is extremely unusual for a physician at an academic institution, almost 10 years after graduation, to leave his home university and go to a different university for graduate-level education. Most physicians tend to stay inside their academic home institutions or rotate only to affiliated hospitals. This doctor's decision was very surprising to me, to his colleagues, and to his boss, and it shows the power of the summer camp experience to change attitudes and behavior.

Continuous Effort to Improve

What we learned when the benefits of the summer camp faded was that we would have to find ways of sustaining the initial energy spawned by the summer camp experience. We tried again and again to make the summer camp better. For example, in the third year we changed the style of education, reducing the number of unidirectional and didactic lectures, and increasing the number of sessions for small-group learning. For example, after a didactic session on study design, we gave the students a scenario including a research question. Their task was to discuss what type of research design to use to answer that specific research question; that is, cohort study, case-control study, and so on. This definitely changed the atmosphere and promoted collaboration among the students, making them feel less competitive and isolated. With this small success, we then changed the format of the presentations on the final day, from individual presentations to group presentations. This made the whole class more dynamic, and the students helped each other to learn and to create a good research plan. This also had a very good long-term effect. Specifically, it became easier to sustain the summer camp's effect, as each member tried to encourage other members of the same group to continue learning, planning, and doing research.

I also tried to give various other opportunities to the summer camp alumni. For example, the foundation that supported the DOPPS offered young clinicians in Japan a chance to do secondary analyses of the Japan-DOPPS data, and I encouraged students to apply for access to those data and do that kind of research. The alumnus who came to Kyoto University for further study of clinical epidemiology at the School of Public Health successfully completed the MCR program, and entered the PhD program. He even said that he would like to study abroad, with the group in Michigan that organized the international DOPPS project, and I encouraged him to do that.

Signs of Improvement

Very slowly but steadily, the number of publications from alumni of the summer camp increased. The doctor who came to Kyoto University for the PhD program did go to study in the United States, where he survived, thrived, and started publishing original articles in first-class international peer-reviewed journals such as *Kidney International* and the *Clinical Journal of the American Society of Nephrology*.

His brave decision to come to Kyoto University and to study abroad stimulated other alumni and summer camp students. Every year, one or two alumni started coming to Kyoto University's MCR program. This became a tradition and by now it has created several "generations" of serious learners from among the summer camp alumni. Since then, the velocity of publications in international peer-reviewed journals has doubled and tripled. The number of presentations at international scientific conferences has also increased. At prominent international meetings (American Society of Nephrology, European Dialysis and Transplantation Association), some summer camp alumni were given awards for their work, such as "best abstract at the meeting."

These successes stimulated other alumni outside Kyoto University, and there was more and more activity and interaction among alumni. To date, there have been more than 100 publications of original articles in international peer-reviewed journals (*see* Figure 6.1). The summer camp has become known and has developed a good reputation among clinical nephrologists in Japan. Many people did not expect this summer camp to last more than three years, but it has now lasted more than eight years and it seems set to continue.

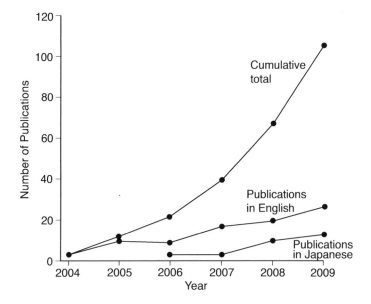

FIGURE 6.1 Publications by nephrologists who had participated in the research-design summer camp

Sustaining Change

In 2011 the number of summer camp alumni reached close to 100, and we decided that the camp should enter a new phase. In this new phase we focus on maintaining, supporting, and extending our accomplishments.

First, like all young researchers, summer camp alumni need help with funding, so I started a program to fund their research projects. I think this funding mechanism is unique. It is partly direct and partly indirect. The indirect funding is about half of the total. It is not really money, but rather a voucher. Groups that receive vouchers can exchange them for services from a non-profit research institute. For example, with two vouchers, a group can "purchase" support for writing a research protocol, for three vouchers they can get statistical consultation, and so on.

Second, we started a short course for director-level clinicians, individuals who are in their forties and are in a position to supervise summer camp alumni. They were never trained in clinical research and some of them are eager to learn its principles and skills. Because they are extremely busy, we decided on a two-day rather than a one-week program. It has been extremely successful. We believe that the two-day program promotes understanding and collaboration between these upper-level clinicians and the summer camp alumni.

We have also created another program for larger numbers of participants – about 200 instead of 12. The main goal of this program is to increase awareness and interest in clinical research among young doctors. Furthermore, we decided to select summer camp participants from among those in the larger group. This creates further motivation since members of the larger group understand that they are among those eligible for selection to attend the summer camp.

Looking back over the past eight years, it is clear that, in addition to publications of original research, summer camp has created quite a few future leaders of clinical nephrology in Japan. Some of them have already risen to the level of associate professor at academic institutions. To some extent, we believe we have achieved our long-term goal of creating a new community of clinical researchers in Japan. I look forward to the 10th anniversary of this summer camp, which will be in 2013.

As rewarding as our results to date are, we still face challenges. For example, our achievements are not yet self-sustaining, and we also need to resolve the problems that we found when we surveyed the MCR-program graduates who had returned to practice in their communities. Trying to find a solution, I discovered that those MCR-program graduates and the summer camp alumni face similar challenges. Specifically, they do not have enough time or support to collect the data that they need to answer their research questions. I took this challenge very seriously, and found a way for our alumni to overcome this barrier.

My goal was to use information technology for a specific purpose: to collect and organize data for clinical researchers outside academia. I applied for and received a three-year grant to develop a system that is small, fast, and cheap, but can still address the unmet needs of clinical researchers. I knew that insurance-claim data could be useful, first, because in Japan these data are now almost all in electronic form, and, second, because they hold information on diagnosis, utilization of laboratory tests, images, drugs, and procedures. What insurance-claim data lack is information on patient outcomes (death and other important events, test results, etc.). The new system, which can be installed on a small server, stores both insurance-claim data and laboratory test results. For outcomes other than test results, such as admission to other hospitals due to adverse events, or death outside a hospital, researchers still need to collect data on their own.

My team created this system within three years. A pilot test in several hospitals was successful. For example, if a clinician were to use data from five years of medical records to answer a particular research question without our new system, retrieving all the data that might be useful and then sorting it and sifting through it to extract only those data that are relevant to the research question would take at least a week. In contrast, with our new system it would take only half an hour. The new system is not fully automated, but it definitely reduces the burden on clinicians who want to identify patients for research and collect only the necessary data, but only have limited time to do so. We hope that it will solve some of the problems faced by alumni from the summer camp and the MCR program. We think this is just a small development, but Kyoto University considers it to be an important innovation, and we were asked to take legal steps to apply for a patent and to transfer the intellectual-property rights to the university.

The next step for us is networking among alumni who do research. A good network is one that is feasible, sustainable, and self-sufficient (not dependent on external funding). I think this is realistic. The network I am planning will have four characteristics, as follows.

1. Network participants will be motivated clinicians who are enthusiastic and who have never-ending research questions. They join the network bringing with them the research literacy that they acquired at the summer camp or in the MCR program. As described above each department at an academic institution in Japan has only one professor, who is also the head of the department and has tremendous power over his (usually not "her") faculty members,

graduate students, and clinicians at the university hospital. In fact, that power extends to clinicians at external, affiliated hospitals. In this top-down system, clinicians outside academia are expected to provide clinical data for large-scale studies that benefit the professor, not to answer their own research questions. I envision a "virtual institution" network in which the "grass-roots" participants are welcome to raise their own research questions. They are not mere data-providers but are its central players. This is what keeps them motivated.

2. This will be a network of empowered life-long learners and particularly clinician-researchers. They will already have been exposed to the basic principles, knowledge, and skills of clinical research at the summer camp and in the MCR program, and their membership in the network will provide continuing motivation for continued learning in clinical epidemiology, biostatistics, meta-analysis, qualitative research methods, and so on.

3. The network will benefit from the information-technology system described above, which will allow efficient extraction of relevant data from vast libraries of medical records. Using this innovation, researchers will not have to spend time sifting through records to collect data while they are engaged in daily clinical practice.

4. The network will evolve. Innovation should continue so that it will become more sophisticated, efficient, and, most important of all, responsive to researchers' needs.

I do not expect this research network to be perfect, but compared with existing structures in Japan, I expect that it will prove to be better for clinical researchers and, ultimately, better for patients. I expect it to keep evolving.

Acknowledgments

I thank Drs. Takahiro Higashi, Yasuaki Hayashino, Shin Yamazaki, Takeo Nakayama, Takashi Kawamura, Yuichi Imanaka, Koji Kawakami, Toshiaki Furukawa, and other faculty members who worked with me in founding and sustaining the MCR program at Kyoto University. I also thank all members of iHope International for supporting the summer camp. I am grateful to Mr. Christopher Holmes for proofreading this chapter, to Drs. Richard Frankel and Thomas Inui for refining it, and to Ms. Misako Nishida for transcribing the dictation on which it is based.

7

Sparking and Sustaining the Essential Functions of Research

Cultivating "Research Mind" – Reason, Dreams, and Discovery

Richard B. Gunderman

Richard Gunderman's Story of a Success in Science: Re-discovering the Power of Love

One of the patients that I have known the very best since I came to work at Riley (Children's) Hospital was a very sick young man with a severe and undiagnosed neurologic condition. He died on Valentine's Day 2012 at the age of 23. I'd known him since he was 14 and also got to know his family well. His parents had six biological children and had adopted many others. When he died on Valentine's Day, I got a call from them asking whether I could say something at his memorial service. I was sick myself at the time but that invitation seemed a real opportunity to try to put into 15 minutes of words what I knew of this family, how they felt about this boy's life, the good that came from it, the burden it represented, and the enduring lessons his life offered – though he himself couldn't intentionally impart any of the lessons. A lot of people looked askance at this young man's life. Some of his health-care team looked on his life as unnecessary, unjustified, and potentially inappropriate. They thought we had done too much for too long to keep his heart beating and that no good was coming of it. It was a great expense to the hospital and to the taxpayers of the State of Indiana. "Poured the dollars down the drain," you could say, because this kid was never going to graduate from college. He'd never go to high school. He couldn't go to kindergarten. He would never hold a paying job. He couldn't feed himself or handle his own toileting. He couldn't sit up in bed. He was completely helpless, essentially devoid of any intentional activity and utterly dependent on others for everything that kept him alive.

It was a service at the New Hope Center, St. Vincent's Hospital. This boy hadn't done good or evil, but somehow the fact he almost "wasn't there" made the love that the people in his life who devoted themselves around the clock to his care all the more visible and breathtaking. In that little service I alluded to the fact that Valentine's Day is a day dedicated to love. I think that's ultimately the lesson of his life. It is love, a deeper kind of love than infatuation or romantic attraction, a feeling that keeps giving even when to most of us it looks like it's pure hurt. I had a chance to try to put those observations into words as a fourth-rate poet – to say that people can still find something precious in a fragile, brittle life. I had had a chance for a time to look at that life through their eyes. On a very occasional basis, at my best moments, because of this experience I can see something in a situation I wouldn't have seen before and I'm immensely grateful. I'll remember that memorial service for a long time and be grateful for the chance I had to participate.

At the center of every person's existence is a dream.

G. K. Chesterton

The chemical structure of benzene had perplexed many of the world's great scientists for years. A natural component of crude oil and one of the most common petrochemicals known to man, benzene had been first isolated by the great British physicist and chemist Michael Faraday in 1825. By the mid-19th century, its chemical formula, composed of six carbon atoms and six hydrogen atoms, had been known for decades, but the rules governing chemical bonding made it difficult to explain how each carbon atom could be bonded to one or two carbon atoms and only a single hydrogen atom. A linear model of benzene simply didn't make sense. Other chemists had suggested that multiple double bonds might be involved. It was in 1865 that the German chemist Friedrich Kekulé published a paper proposing that benzene was not a linear molecule but a ring whose carbon atoms were linked by alternating single and double bonds.

Kekulé later described his discovery of the ring structure of benzene as having occurred to him in a dream. He had been working on the problem for many years, without success. Then one day he was sitting by the fire, daydreaming, when before his eyes appeared a pair of serpents. The serpents opened their mouths and caught each other's tails, creating a ring. This led Kekulé to the sudden realization that benzene might be hexagonal. The structure had never appeared on the chalkboards of chemists who had been trying to deduce it by the laws of logic, and it was utterly unlike anything else in chemistry. In this remarkable anecdote, Kekulé reveals that science does not always progress strictly by the link-by-link construction of chains of logic. In many cases, what is needed is a moment of inspiration, a sudden burst of insight whose timing is hard to predict and whose source is impossible to pinpoint. Above all, what is needed is the capacity to dream.

From a psychological point of view, dreams play a vital role in human life. The rapid eye movement (REM) phase of sleep occupies approximately 60% of our non-waking hours, during which we dream. Complete sleep deprivation is incompatible with life, and less severe forms produce deficits in attention, working memory, and skills such as driving. Of course, human beings are not the only creatures that dream. There is good evidence that other animals such as horses, dogs, and rats dream as well. And experiments with rats appear to demonstrate that dreams play an important role in the consolidation of memory and learning, as though the mind were sorting through the events of the day to determine what is worth retaining. In addition, dreams enable us to discover new associations between recent and remote events, connecting up ideas and experiences in new ways. Dreams also appear to play an important role in creativity, as people who are allowed to sleep after being presented with a problem are more likely to discover innovative solutions.

Dreams are biologically necessary, but few physicians and scientists would suggest that they have a role to play in guiding reason and science. The roots of this scientific suspicion of dreams can be traced in part to the work of Rene Descartes, whose *Discourse on the Method of Rightly Conducting the Reason and Seeking Truth in the Sciences* (1637) posits conscious reason as the only reliable guide. This partly autobiographical treatise contains one of the most famous utterances in the history of philosophy, "I think, therefore I am." In it, Descartes examines human knowledge skeptically, finding that sense perceptions can always deceive us. The sun, for example, must be much larger than it appears when we look at it. Even less reliable are the fantastic images presented to our minds in dreams. On what then can we pin our hopes for certain knowledge? Descartes argues that the only thing we can know with absolute certainty is our own rational thought. To progress, science must do away with mere opinions. Instead we must build our understanding step by step, beginning with the simplest truth – that we think.

Against the Cartesian approach stands the work of Sigmund Freud. In his great treatise, the 1899 *The Interpretation of Dreams*, Freud argues that our mind and thoughts, far from being the clearest and most reliable objects of our aware-ness, are in fact among the very most mysterious. Freud divides the mind into at least two territories, the conscious and the unconscious. The conscious is the part we are aware of, such as our awareness of the steps we are taking in solving a complex mathematical problem. Yet, in Freud's model, consciousness is but the tip of the psychic iceberg. The unconscious, a much larger, non-rational realm of basic biological drives, lies beneath our awareness. The most powerful forces at work in the human psyche lurk in this domain. Much of this territory is not only unknown but unknowable, in part because reason cannot grasp it. To gain any real insight into this realm, we must proceed not by reason, but by dreams. In fact, Freud referred to dreams as the "royal road to the unconscious."

Today we recognize the power of dreams to shape history. Martin Luther King Jr. relied on the metaphor of a dream when he delivered one of the most important speeches of the 20th century standing on the steps of the Lincoln Memorial in Washington DC in August of 1963. King did not say, "I have a logical argument" or "I have a strategic plan." Instead he said, "I have a dream," "I have a dream that my four little children will one day live in a nation where they will be judged not by the color of their skin but by the content of their character." King did not attempt to construct a rational argument that racism is wrong or that all people should enjoy the same liberties and mutual respect. Instead he spoke as a Baptist preacher, invoking articles of faith from the Bible, the Declaration of Independence, the Constitution, and the Emancipation Proclamation. Logic and reason may direct understanding, but the rhetoric of dreams inspires the heart, engaging our highest aspirations.

Freud did students of science and psychology an important service by calling attention to the role of non-rational and often obscure forces in shaping human thought. Dreams have a power among human beings largely denied to the forces of unadulterated reason, as King's speech amply testifies. Yet Freud also did us a profound disservice by structuring his model of the psyche in a way that places the unconscious below the conscious. If dreams originate in the unconscious, as

Freud holds, they necessarily rise up from below, rather than descending upon us from above. In addition, Freud's model suggests that dreams arise entirely from within the psyche, eliminating the possibility that dreams bear insights from outside the self. What if dreams sometimes come to us from above? To explore this possibility, let us turn to a quite different source, one eschewed by Descartes and Freud but cherished by King.

Consider the nature and role of dreams in one of the foundational texts of our civilization, the Book of Genesis. Genesis takes dreams very seriously. In fact, nearly a third of the dream accounts in the entire Bible are found in this book. One particularly notable example is Jacob's dream at Bethel, through which he first receives the divine covenant as well as promises from God about his future and the future of his offspring. Another is the dream in which Jacob wrestles with God, as a result of which he undergoes a transformation in identity. A third example is the dream of Pharaoh concerning the coming famine, which only Joseph can interpret for him. These and other accounts in the Book of Genesis represent some of the most revealing portraits of dreams and their transformative power available to us. By briefly exploring each, we can gain a deeper appreciation for the power of dreams and the role they may play in our professional and personal lives.

To understand Jacob's dream at Bethel, we must see it in context. Jacob has just taken advantage of his older twin brother Esau and deceived his father Isaac in an effort to obtain his father's birthright and blessing, the rights to the greater share of his father's property and the covenant established between his grandfather Abraham and God. He has been sent away by his mother, whom he will never see again, with nothing, to seek refuge from his vengeful brother in the house of his uncle Laban. He is alone in a strange place. Overcome by fatigue, he lays his head down on the only pillow available, a stone. Then he dreams of a ladder bridging the earth and heaven, along which angels are ascending and descending. During the dream, God gives him land, tells him his descendants will be numerous and a blessing to all people, and assures him that he will have divine protection and guidance. When Jacob awakes, he realizes that "God is in this place," makes an altar of the stone, declares that the divinity who has just revealed himself will be his god, and agrees to give him back a tenth of everything he has been given.

Jacob's dream at Bethel offers a number of important insights into the power of dreams. First, in contrast to the Freudian view that sees God and heaven as projections of human desires, Jacob's dream reveals a higher or heavenly realm. What we see around us every day does not represent the full extent of reality.

Moreover, this higher realm can be connected to our everyday experience, permitting human beings to look at life from a higher, more comprehensive, deeper, and longer-term and perhaps even eternal perspective. Seen from this perspective, many of our everyday preoccupations look small, while other concerns loom larger. From his dream Jacob learns that his life is imbued with a significance that he had not known, that he is living not just for himself but for those who came before and those who will follow after him, and that his life and that of his descendants can enrich all mankind. Jacob begins to see his life as serving not primarily himself but God.

Equally transformative insights spring from Jacob's struggle with God. Again, to grasp the meaning of the account, we need to see it in context. Jacob has not seen Esau in 20 years. During this time, he has married, become the father of many children, and acquired property. The last time he and his brother were under the same roof Esau was plotting Jacob's murder in vengeance for Jacob's deception regarding the blessing. On his journey back to Canaan, Jacob is frightened to learn that Esau is approaching him with a force of 400 men. The night before their reunion, a troubled Jacob dreams of wrestling until daybreak with a stranger. The stranger does not overpower him, but touches his hip, causing Jacob to walk with a limp. When it is finished, Jacob demands a blessing and is told that henceforth he shall be known as Israel, "one who struggled with God." Jacob and Esau are then happily reunited.

Before this encounter, Jacob was known by a name that means "supplanter" or perhaps "deceiver." He had deceived his father and supplanted his brother in taking the birthright and blessing that, by tradition and Isaac's estimation, should have gone to Esau. Since then, however, the deceiver has become the deceived and the supplanter the supplanted, as his uncle Laban has cheated him out of seven years' labor and replaced Rachel, the daughter he wished to marry, with another, Leah. Earlier in his life Jacob referred to "my father's God," but now he has lived for 20 years knowing this same God as his own. In the past, he has struggled with men, but now he has struggled with God. As a result, he has become a new man, inspired by a radically transformed notion of what matters most in life. He is no longer the deceiver, but one who has sought to know the truth, seeking to make sense of his life from a divine perspective. His new name reflects this transformation, which has required the span of an entire generation to complete.

The next highly revealing dream involves not Jacob but one of Jacob's sons, Joseph. Joseph is a dreamer, and perhaps partly for this reason he is also his father's favorite of 12 sons. His dreams have earned his brothers' ire and led them to plot to kill him, though they eventually sell him into slavery. While in prison for a crime he did not commit, Joseph correctly interprets the dreams of the Pharaoh's cup bearer and baker. Then Pharaoh has dreams that none of his experts can interpret. The dreams include seven fat cows being devoured by seven lean cows. He turns to Joseph, who offers the interpretation that seven years of agricultural abundance will be followed by seven years of famine, advising Pharaoh that he should store the surplus grain from the abundant years. In gratitude, Pharaoh releases Joseph from prison and makes him his right-hand man, in charge of all the land of Egypt. Eventually, Joseph's starving brothers are sent by their father to Pharaoh to buy grain, leading eventually to a reunion of Joseph and his brothers.

In this account, we learn that dreams may be dangerous and unpleasant. They may bring us together with those we love but they also may alienate us from them. Dreams also sometimes tell us things we would rather not hear, just as Pharaoh's dreams foretell the demise of his baker. And even dreams with the potential to enrich our lives may not reach us as direct commands or promises from the higher realm. They often speak indirectly, in the manner of metaphors or parables that require interpretation. Even the greatest earthly power, Pharaoh, cannot understand his own dreams, nor can his imperial court. Perhaps the leaders are so preoccupied with management and administration of the earthly realm that they cannot understand the heavenly perspective. At any rate, Joseph, favored by God, is able to understand and provide an accurate interpretation. Though an immensely able administrator, Joseph grasps that a higher purpose is at work in human affairs.

What are the lessons of these stories of dreams and dreaming for academic physicians and health science centers? The aspiration to understand the larger order plays an important role in discovery. People who are content with what immediately meets the eye are unlikely to pursue new vistas. Also, such new vistas have a natural tendency to be disruptive. In some cases, edifices must be demolished before new ones can take their place. Space and time are necessary if we are to look at things anew. At a literal level, some physicians get too little sleep, which does not permit sufficient time for dreaming. Others are so busy and occupied with daily work that there is no time to notice dreams, let alone to reflect on them. In a more metaphorical sense, we need to create and sustain organizational contexts where dreaming can take place and people can share their dreams. If every interpersonal interaction takes place in a formal meeting and if every meeting agenda is filled with operational issues, nothing is left for people to step back and muse on larger and ultimately more important questions that can foster transformational creativity. In what activities are we frittering away our careers and lives? What new paths should we be exploring? What might we as an organization aspire to be and do?

There is an old Celtic saying that heaven and earth are only a few feet apart, but in "thin" places that gap becomes narrower still. The notion is that some places open up more possibilities than others for sensing and perhaps even communing with what is most important. Such thin places might include mountain tops, waterfalls, and deep caves. Perhaps Jacob was seeking to mark such a place when he erected the stone at Bethel. And what if places are not the only things that can be thin? What if times, stories, works of art, and people can be thin as well? What if there are ways to make organizations and even particular meetings thinner than they would otherwise be? Can we point to such experiences in the professional and personal spheres of our own lives?

A related notion is that of liminality. The term comes from a Latin root meaning boundary or threshold. As developed in anthropology by Victor Turner and others, liminality refers to a state or condition in which established orders are called into question, when new ways of understanding or acting become possible. Examples include so-called rites of passage, through which girls become women and boys become men. Such rites often involve a period of isolation, during which an individual or group is led to question the previous order before later becoming part of a new one. In this sense, liminal experiences are both destructive and constructive, permitting integration into a new kind or level of order. Thinness and liminality invoke neither the pure waking state nor the pure dream state, but a kind of twilight state, where day and night, darkness and light, encounter one another.

If we grant that the experiences of thinness and liminality have an important role to play in creativity and transformation, what can we do to foster them? The first step is to recognize the importance of experiences that leave us asking, "Did that really happen?" The next is to put ourselves in situations where normal structures can no longer be taken for granted. For example, we might do away with clocks for a time, set aside titles and hierarchies, and ask people to tell stories or create works of art, without any express focus on the pressing problems of work or personal life. To get to some place new, whether a new vista or a new insight, we need to pass through unfamiliar territory, which involves a certain degree of disorientation and even discomfort. Finally, we need to bear in mind that often the goal is not to enter a liminal state on a merely individual basis, but to achieve some measure of shared liminal experience.

The idea that we do not generate twilight experiences such as dreams ourselves, that instead they come to us from elsewhere, is an important one. The ancient Greeks invoked the muses, female deities who represented the source of inspiration, from whose name we get the word "music." At the beginning of his two great epics, the *Iliad* and *Odyssey*, Homer invokes the muses, praying that they will sing through him. Both the ancient Greeks and the ancient Hebrews believed in theophanies, experiences where a divinity appears to a human being, often during sleep. When the god speaks, we learn things we did not know. We learn to look again in new ways at things we long ago ceased to notice. And we undergo transformations. Jacob makes the god of his father his own, and it is during such a theophany that he is transformed from Jacob into Israel. It is ironic that it takes a dream to awaken us from our slumber and show us what is really going on.

There is another lesson to be gleaned from Jacob's dreams, both of which occur when he is alone in the desert at night. It is often when we are in the dark, isolated and discouraged, that we gain the deepest insights into our own character and the purposes of our work and life. When everything is going along swimmingly, there seems to be little cause to pause and reflect. But when we have suffered a setback, where our assumptions and expectations have been challenge or disappointed, or when accustomed relationships have been disrupted, we begin asking different kinds of questions. The Greeks said that wisdom comes only through suffering. Whether this is literally true or not, it is certainly the case that some of our most important insights are born of disappointment and despair, when we switch to a new line of research, move to a new position, or discover a new calling in life. It is possible that setbacks in research such as a failed grant or a long-term collaboration that dissolves, forcing re-thinking and adoption of new perspectives or methods may serve as a spur to innovation. As the Chinese have observed, "crisis" is a combination of "risk" and "opportunity." We should be careful never to let disappointments go to waste.

Such reminders are necessary because, as physicians, scientists, and administrators, we sometimes exhibit a tendency to avoid the novel. We have been born and bred to know the answers, and it can be difficult to admit to ourselves, let alone others, that we do not know. We treasure certainty, and find uncertainty difficult to bear. We like to think that life is entirely reasonable, and that it should be possible to navigate through our personal and professional lives in strictly logical terms. We dread the unexpected, and like to be in control at all times. Hence it is perfectly natural for us to avoid situations where we are in the dark, alone, uncertain about what is going on or how to proceed, and feeling that we are not in control. Yet it is precisely when we dream that we are able to see anew. Checklists help us get routine work done efficiently and with low rates of error, but they are of no value when it comes to creativity and insight. In fact, they may prove positively counterproductive.

To lead effectively, we need to be prepared to relinquish our managerial prerogatives. We need to set aside our worldly cares and desires to predict and control everything that happens. We cannot manage our dreams, because they come to us unbidden and proceed according to their own initiative. If we programmed every moment of our day, how could we possibly achieve truly novel insights? To open ourselves up to dreams requires that we open ourselves up and accept our vulnerability. Not only are we not in control, we do not even understand what is happening. This is why interpretation is needed. Dreams operate at multiple levels. The last thing we should say to ourselves or others is, "That will never work here," or "Are you crazy?" Dreams open up new visions of what we know, who we are, and who we can become, both individually and collectively. We need to foster conditions in which our eyes can be opened to larger realities and possibilities than the ones we have learned or been taught to take for granted.

8

The Relationship-Centered Care Research Network

Its Birth, Life-cycle and Lessons Learned Along the Way

Richard M. Frankel, Penelope R. Williamson, Dana Gelb Safran, Debra Roter, and The Relationship-Centered Care Research Network: Mary Catherine Beach, Howard Beckman, Lisa A. Cooper, Judith A. Hall, Paul Haidet, Thomas S. Inui, William L. Miller, David L. Mossbarger, and Howard F. Stein

> ### Richard Frankel's Story of a Success in Science: Teaching Each Other the Fundamentals of the Game as Researchers and Friends
>
> Early in my career I met a general internist, Howard Beckman, and we got to know one another by playing racquetball. He had played lacrosse for Brandeis, and I got to college on a track scholarship. I was fast but my hand-eye coordination was not very good. Howard's hand-eye coordination was excellent so he would routinely beat me ... 15–0, 15–1 ... and one day he said this can't be very much fun. I said, "No, I'm having a good time. It's a good workout." He said, "Let me teach you the fundamentals of the game." He gave me some exercises to do when we weren't playing competitively. I would practice those fundamentals and my game improved. I was still losing but I was losing much more competitively. This was in Detroit. I had moved from Boston to Detroit which itself is a story of moving from feeling

very successful to initially feeling quite unsuccessful because Detroit was not on my top 115 cities I wanted to settle in. I had training in microanalysis and conversation analysis. I had lots of technical expertise but I had never really worked in a medical setting. Howard and I decided to work together. We studied the opening of the medical encounter, using 74 videotapes of residents in our residency program. We would get together after work on our own time without any funding and we just started looking at the tapes. It was actually a pretty crowded field even in the 1980s. When we started our work we followed a naturalist qualitative research design – to see what we could observe without making any assumptions about what is observable. Howard brought a strong clinical sense, because that was the work he did and he wasn't schooled in sociology or social psychology. The chemistry between us worked out well. The publication from this work has become a classic in the field, and I think this was partially because we were working from substantially different perspectives. We weren't starting where others had stopped, but we were taking a fresh approach. In February 1984, we submitted the paper to the *Annals of Internal Medicine*, which seemed like a really big stretch for what we were doing. I got a call from Howard saying the paper had been provisionally accepted. It felt right for a number of reasons. It felt right because it was the introduction of a direct observation method that I think had been missing until then. It felt right to me because it was an application of an approach I had used before but never in a clinical context. It felt right because it grew out of our blood, sweat, and tears of just looking and seeing what we could see. It's a paper based on 74 cases and yet, some 30-odd years later, it's cited as a classic in the field, and there have been several follow-up studies that have validated our findings that we came up with. The critical element was working in a partnership, a highly functional partnership.

Introduction

"Keeping considerations of self and professional together permits us to see work as an expression of self, and professional aspirations for trustworthiness and virtuous action as aspirations of our own heart. In a field that demands as much of us as medicine, anything less than

this integration of person and professional may be unsupportable in the long run."

— Thomas Inui[2]

"In the real world of scientific clinical investigators, the Relationship-centered Research Network was our Camelot."

— RCCRN, Participant E

In his short story "The Loneliness of the Long Distance Runner,"[1] Alan Sillitoe uses long-distance running as a metaphor for how one succeeds in life. The message of the narrative is that if one is willing to sacrifice physically, mentally, and spiritually, and at the same time concentrate on a single outcome, success is possible if one wants it badly enough. After rigorously training for and leading in a race that could result in his freedom from a juvenile detention center, Colin, the protagonist in Sillitoe's narrative, stops just short of the finish line, allowing a competitor to win. The implication of the character's motivation to win, and choice to lose, is clear. Success and choices in life are solitary and hard-won.

Sillitoe's metaphor of individual sacrifice, singular focus and hard work applies in equal measure to traditional thinking about how to achieve success in a research career. Competition for promotion and tenure, grant dollars and peer-reviewed publication is fierce and despite calls for collaboration and multi-disciplinary work individual performance metrics are still the coin of the realm in many academic health science centers. For many, a research career is a long, lonely path. Where collaboration does occur, it is often based on instrumental rather than interpersonal goals and the main objective, sometimes the only objective, is "getting the work done at all costs." As Inui notes above, however, the traditional formula for success may neither be possible nor desirable for training medical professionals, especially physicians, for a lifetime of service. Our question for this chapter is, "What happens when instrumental and interpersonal goals are merged in the context of collaborative *research?"*

The narrative that follows describes an experiment in forming a relationship-centered research network. Its birth and life-cycle were based on attention to doing good science and at the same time retaining, building, and sustaining strong interpersonal relationships and a sense of community. We begin by describing the background of the Relationship-Centered Care Initiative (RCCI) and one of its arms, the Relationship-Centered Care Research Network (RCCRN), the intentional process that was used to create community, the settings in which the network met, how theoretical and methodological differences were experienced, the role of the external facilitator, funding, and the work products of the network.

In writing this chapter, we have relied upon artifacts, such as progress and final reports and planning and personal notes from each of the network's face-to-face meetings. In addition, the authors used an iterative consensus-building process to develop an in-depth interview guide addressing questions of interest.[3] Between April and August of 2011, two of the authors, PW and RMF, conducted phone or in-person interviews with each of the network members. (*See* Appendix 1 for a list of questions used in the interviews.) Field notes and transcriptions were used to identify emergent themes using an immersion/crystallization approach.[4] Finally, a member check was done by sending drafts of the chapter to each network member for their review and comment.

Background

Planning for the Relationship-Centered Care Initiative began in the spring of 2001 with the two co-principal investigators who conceived of a project that would involve two arms: (1) applying Relationship-Centered Care principles to changing the culture of a large medical school[5,6] and (2) creating a relationship-centered care research network. The project was funded by the Fetzer Institute of Kalamazoo, Michigan.

The Relationship-Centered Care Research Network was conceptualized as an opportunity to bring together a diverse group of highly successful senior and junior researchers whose work was considered synergistic with principles of relationship-centered care that had been articulated a decade earlier in a jointly sponsored Pew/Fetzer monograph on health professions education.[7] Relationship-Centered Care focuses on the dynamic interplay and influence of communication and relationship on processes and outcomes of care.[7] One of the PIs for the parent RCCI project (TSI) had led the taskforce; the other PI (RF), and the co-PI for the RCCN (DR), had also been members of the taskforce.

Although there was overall alignment with RCC principles among those invited to participate, we sought diversity in age, gender, professional background, and methodological orientation. Invitations to join a network of well-established and junior researchers interested in RCC were sent to 10 individuals in North America. The invitation outlined the time commitment (8–9 face-to-face meetings over 3–4 years, collaborative research projects, presentations, and scholarly products such as publications) and general expectations for the network's functioning. Nine of the 10 invitees agreed to participate; one individual's schedule would not permit participation. Both the principal investigators are health services researchers and their participation brought the group size to 11.

In the initial planning process we reasoned that it would be useful to embody the principles of relationship-centered care in building the research network. Since the group was composed of a diverse set of individuals, some of whom had worked together and others who were strangers to one another, we decided to invite an outside facilitator (PW) who was skilled in small group formation and was also involved in the second arm of the RCC initiative to join the effort. A design team was created, consisting of the two PIs for the project, our external consultant (PW), and one researcher from the network (DR and, later, DGS). The design team met before each meeting to plan and assess progress in the network.

The First Face-to-Face Meeting

The RCCRN had its first day-and-a-half-long, face-to-face meeting at the home of one of the participants in September of 2003, and its ninth, and last, face-to-face meeting in November of 2007. During its four years, this group of highly productive researchers with interests in clinician–patient communication came together to identify common interests and conduct research. The formal research agenda was focused on relationship-centered communication in health care – including not only clinician-to-patient, but the full range of other relationships involved among colleagues, administrators, patients, and families. At the same time an intention was set to use a formation process[8] to create a sense of community among the researchers and explore what differences, if any, working in this way had on the quality and content of the research.

Eleven researchers, our external facilitator, a project manager, and a representative from the Fetzer Institute attended the first meeting. Some of the goals for the first meeting were a little unusual for a group of high-profile researchers and included the idea that by the end of the meeting participants would, in addition to focusing on technical aspects of relationship-centered care research, "Begin to think of themselves as a community and network with a common purpose." In order to achieve this goal, a community-building formation exercise was planned. It consisted of inviting each group member to pair off with another and recall a high-point research experience, ". . . in which you were working with others in a trustworthy environment where each person was able to share ideas openly, where you felt connected to your values, excited by the work, able to show up fully and to bring your gifts to bear."

After each pair had shared their stories with one another the whole group gathered to hear each person tell their partner's story with the goal of identifying common themes and facilitators of doing research in community. The themes that emerged informed subsequent topics on the agenda: current thinking about relationship-centered care, developing an outline for a white paper on the state of the science of RCC, generating a list of exciting topics that network members were interested in exploring, and the implications of key decisions such as when and where to meet for subsequent meetings, whether to work in teams or as individuals, and when to host a national meeting to share and discuss findings.

Participants' Recollections of the First Meeting

More than seven years have passed since the first face-to-face meeting. We were interested in knowing what participants recalled about their first experiences with the network. One question asked of all participants was, "Please recall the evening of our first gathering as a group. What stands out for you from that meeting? As you think about other research collaborations that you have participated in, was there anything unusual or different that you noticed about the beginning of the RCCRN initiative?" Responses varied from "vague memories," to a detailed description of the community-building portion of the meeting.

Several themes were prominent in the responses. The first was that, unlike many research meetings where there is an emphasis on accomplishing tasks, the RCCRN network began by bringing people into relationship in a personal way. This theme is well illustrated by a quote from participant "B" who said, "I remember that we had an exercise [an icebreaker] where we took the question and went and asked everybody and then tried to remember their answers, or wrote them down . . . We didn't come together with any apparent research agenda. I mean, it wasn't the first thing that happened, whereas with most research meetings, there is an agenda related to a research project." Participant "C" said, "I remember the facilitator with her hokey exercises [which] were useful in the end. I'm a task-oriented person. Being immersed in the moment with smart people who were not competing turned out to be wonderful." A variation of this theme was echoed by participant "G," who focused on what it was like to enter the group for the first time. "I remember walking up the back steps and into the kitchen – a lot of activity . . . [a group dinner was being prepared] and it felt like being at a party at someone's house except I didn't really know anyone. It felt kind of scary in a way (cocktail party feeling) if you don't know a soul. Don't know what to say. – Hung out in back yard. I really remember the ice breaker activity and LOVED IT and the questions that were used. I also remember the first conversation seated around the living room . . . and trading stories and telling each other's stories – all of that is really vivid."

By design, there were differences in professional degrees (MD/PhD/Dr. PH, ScD), age, and career stage in the network. Some of the challenges of these differences were reflected in recollections of the first meeting. For example, participant "F," a senior member of the group, commented, "At the first meeting we had to talk to another person. I talked to [one of the junior faculty] and I had a difficult time not thinking of her as a daughter. It was a very odd feeling. I had to work at it over the next month – to think of her as a colleague, not a daughter. I was really surprised." Another participant, "K," described his surprise at meeting researchers whose work was familiar but whom he had not met face to face. "What I recall from the first meeting was these images of some of the researchers that I didn't know from before as being super human. And, 'wow' I discovered that they're human just like me!"

A final theme was that of parallel process, the idea that a fundamental understanding of Relationship-Centered Care could be discovered in the group's own processes and experiences. This theme was captured by participant "E," who asserted, ". . . you [the facilitators] established from the outset, a certain format in which check-ins (offering an invitation to each person of reflecting on how they are doing at the moment or what might be going on for them outside of the meeting that might be diverting their attention) always had to come before tasks. And the check-ins set the stage for getting the work done, so we were persons first, with how we felt that day and what we were bringing to it, and that sort of thing which took seriously our own work relationships, so relationship-centered care began at home."

Setting

Early on in the network's development a decision was made to meet in members' homes rather than in university or medical school facilities. In fact, the first planning meeting of the leadership group was held in the home of one of the co-principal investigators (TSI). The decision that the entire group would meet informally, however, was serendipitous and motivated by a practical concern for the first group meeting – the host's spouse was traveling and she had child care responsibilities at home. As she reflected, ". . . when we talked through how different it would feel to welcome these people as if we were bringing them together in a home rather than into a hotel, it seemed to me that it made complete sense." With the exception of one meeting, which occurred in a hotel in Chicago and took advantage of the fact that almost all network members were attending a professional meeting, all face-to-face meetings occurred in "personal" spaces, often inhabited by spouses, children, pets, and sometimes neighbors.

Curious to know what effect(s) the decision to meet in an informal setting had on network members, we asked in the interviews, "Early on we decided to meet in people's homes rather than in institutional settings. What difference(s) if any did the change in venue make for you personally? In terms of group formation?" Universally, network members praised the decision to meet in an informal setting and described their reactions. For some participants this had an impact in terms of developing and sustaining meaningful long-term relationships. For example, participant "C" reflected, "Meeting in people's homes is what allowed the personal connections to develop. A lot of meetings I go to are held in hotels, restaurants, etc., and few of the connections I make in these meetings end up being substantial or long-term." Participant "B" echoed this theme in asserting, ". . . not only do you see what kind of furniture people pick out, what they hang on their walls but I think that your orientation toward work is different when you're in a home because it's not common that you're doing work with other people in someone's home, or your own home, so you tend to think of it a little bit more as a relationship kind of place to be." Participant "K" agreed and went on to assert that "Meeting in a place where we started with the humanization of who we all are and where disruptions of all sorts occur, children show up, phone calls come in, shrinks the egos and creates the common field that we all share, that we've all stumbled in and lived through and shared. We see each other as equal in our humanity."

Geographically, network members came from as far West and Southwest as Oklahoma and Texas as well as from the Midwest and Northeast. Meetings were held in cities where travel was most convenient for the largest number of participants. As a result, meetings were held in Baltimore (where four network members resided), Boston (where two members resided) and Indianapolis (where three members resided). For those whose homes were gathering sites the meetings had particular meaning. For instance, participant "G" noted, "When we were in MY home it was the most delicious thing. One of the things that gives me the greatest joy in my life is to have my home humming with people, ideas and conversation. To have had that with this group of people, multiple times, is something I'll always treasure. . . . Our being in others' homes contributed to people's willingness to engage in a more reflective way than being in an institutional setting. The informal setting, moving back and forth between the personal and the professional, allowed the conversations to move forward and felt very natural." At least one participant, "C," felt that *not* meeting in her home was a missed opportunity. For this participant, home had a special cultural relevance. "I always wished I could have hosted a meeting at my home too so that others in the network could get to know who I am more . . . I come from quite a different culture from many people in the group and it would have allowed me to share a lot of that."

Several participants noted that even when the meeting was in a hotel, the ease of relationships that had already been established prevailed. This observation was nicely summarized by participant "E" who asserted, "It felt "hamish" (Yiddish slang for cozy or inviting) in the sense that the informality that allowed you to get up and get a bagel, or go to the bathroom or get coffee, in the middle of actual work, that relationship stuff pervaded the atmosphere and facilitated getting the work done. It's interesting, that there was one exception, the meeting in that strange back room in Chicago, and I got the feeling that even though it was a little stiffer than meeting in homes I could bring that feeling and sensibility of our relationships into that very awkward, structured room. So, for me, the acid test was when we got out of the element of being in people's homes I could transpose the homey feeling from where we had been before to this, to this awkward place and it wasn't as awkward as it could have been."

In summary, there was unanimity that the setting of members' homes was conducive to deeper, long-lasting relationships that facilitated the work of the group. In fact, nurturing and sustaining these relationships became a core value. The effect was strong enough so that even when the group met in a more formal meeting space, they were able to seamlessly transform it into one that was aligned with an informal style that had become a group value.

Differences in Theoretical and Methodological Outlook

By design, the research network included individuals with different professional and methodological orientations. The group included representatives from internal medicine, family medicine, psychology, health services research, anthropology/sociology, and public health. In terms of methodological approaches, the group contained both qualitative and quantitative researchers with further divisions into subspecialties such as conversation analysis, ethnographic field analysis, narrative analysis, epidemiology, experimental design, outcomes-based interventions, and quantitative interaction analysis. Many of these differences were well-known historically and some, such as tensions between quantitative and qualitative communication researchers, had appeared in the literature. Such differences had the potential to split the group and make working together difficult.

We were interested to know, in retrospect, how network members experienced the diversity in the group and asked, "There were a number of strong professional differences (theory, method, funding, etc.) that marked the group. What was your experience of those differences at the beginning of the initiative?" Overwhelmingly, network members stated that they didn't really attend to the differences, except as an opportunity to learn. For instance, participant "A" stated, "I was someone who hoped and expected to learn and valued the disciplinary differences and even the disputation that came from that as a source of learning." Likewise, participant "D" noticed differences and saw them as adding to the group's dialogs. She stated, "Some folks were more into organizational work, some more into the health system side of things; a few more in humanities (philosophy, art and psychology, liberal arts orientation) and then those more in medicine and in academic medicine/public health. I just noticed they were there and brought more richness to our conversations and perspectives." Participant "F" asserted, "Everyone in the group was interested in exploring. It was not clubby, inclusionary or exclusionary."

Others, such as participant "E," noted the lack of ego and potential use of power, prestige, and authority in the group process. "I felt very good professionally and relationally from the outset. I did not feel any professional posturing . . . I did not feel leadership posturing or self-aggrandizement for creating infantilizing dependency; instead, you created a mature work group dependency. It was so refreshing." In complementary fashion, but focusing on awareness of what was present rather than what was absent, participant "B" noted, "I don't know that I thought very much about a difference in methodological approaches. What I noticed was a difference in personal orientation toward, sort of right-brain, left-brain orientations within the group. And so it's not true and it's not fair to say that qualitative is one quantitative is the other, so I wouldn't necessarily match them to that. But I think it was more differences in the kind of people that were there, versus, say, approaches that they might apply to the work. For example, I noticed that there were some people who seemed more comfortable with silence, more comfortable with strong emotion and others who didn't want that as much, or that wasn't their go-to way of being."

One of the major concerns the organizers had in forming the RCCRN was the diversity of the group in terms of age, gender, professional training, and theoretical and methodological orientation. As it turned out, network members focused less on differences that might divide the group and its work, and more on the unique contributions different voices made to the network's overall effort and output. This outcome is perhaps one strong indicator of the group's having formed and acted together as a community of purpose rather than a collection of individuals competing for control of intellectual and/or economic resources.

The Role of an External Facilitator

While the decision to meet in network members' homes was serendipitous, the idea of asking an outside facilitator to help create community was not. We retained the services of Penny Williamson ScD, an internationally well-known small group facilitator who was engaged in the arm of the overall relationship-centered care initiative that was simultaneously taking place at the Indiana University School of Medicine under the same leadership as the RCCRN.

Penny defined her role as introducing formation principles as a way of building a community and network with a common purpose. To that end, she used a number of facilitation practices such as appreciative check-in and debrief to begin and end each meeting, paired interviews, poetry, journaling, walkabouts, and silent times for reflection during meetings. We asked network members to reflect on ways in which her presence affected the group and its functioning and whether there were specific moments of facilitation which were particularly meaningful.

As might be expected from someone whose role was by design in the background creating the conditions for a community to emerge and thrive, several members only had vague memories of her activities. For example, participant "G" stated, "The group formation part I don't remember very well. I was oblivious to the intentions of the leaders and new to the group. As a result I didn't take in a lot of what was happening. I remember the first meeting and the first exercise that Penny put together. I was impressed, thought it was cool and meaningful; then, her quiet steady presence pulled us forward and kept us going." A similar sentiment was voiced by participant "J" who said, "Penny provided a little bit of guiding force, helped us have more structure to the process." Similarly, participant

"B" stated, "I have more of an emotional feeling, a warm feeling about Penny's presence than I have a particular memory of it."

Others felt that Penny had a larger influence on the group and its direction. For instance, participant "A" stated, "[Penny] gave everyone the confidence there was kind of a process management intelligence at work and that there would be a possibility that we could relax into that, maybe take a few more risks but be assured that all voices would be heard." Participant "B" asserted, "Well, I don't know what would have happened without Penny. I mean, Penny set the tone for the meetings and it's possible, maybe, that somebody else could have done that, but they never tried it."

Not every participant felt satisfied or comfortable with the facilitator's style. For example, participant "C" found it, ". . . a bit too sugary sometimes but it did keep a tone. Also, it went painfully slowly at first, but modeled the way it was intended to go." Another participant, "H," stated, "I'm not sure that I think her facilitation made that much of a difference. If I had some resistance, it was to her structuring because there was this assumption that this is the way the group will go and to be truthful there were times when I felt a little manipulated. . . . I think Penny did do a great job. It's more about how I respond to things, so, you know, I do have a lot of resistance to stuff like the poetry thing. You know, sometimes I felt annoyed. And sometimes it was hard to remind myself how hard she was working and how useful it was to the process, but that still didn't take away that feeling of being, I guess manipulated is what keeps coming to my mind."

It is clear from participants' comments that having an external facilitator allowed the group to think and act together which was consistent with one of the goals of the initiative, to create community as a resource for conducting Relationship-Centered Care research. Several participants stated that they couldn't imagine how the group could have accomplished its goals without a facilitator to manage the process and keep things moving. And, although memories of specific moments of facilitation tended to be indistinct among members, the feeling tone (being in a safe space, knowing someone was monitoring the process, and so on) was very much in evidence. Although there was overall praise for her facilitation, two members felt as though facilitation of the group made little difference and could have been omitted.

The Role of Others Supporting the Project

Logistic support and day-to-day management of the project fell to the project manager, Dave Mossbarger. As well, a representative of the Fetzer Institute, Dave Sluyter, attended several of the face-to-face meetings. We were interested in knowing how the group experienced these individuals and asked, "In addition to the researchers and facilitator there were other members of the group including the project manager and a representative from Fetzer. From your perspective what role did they play in your experience of the initiative?"

Participant G summarized the project manager's impact by stating, "Dave Mossbarger was this incredibly helpful presence – just unassuming, ready to be of service at every turn and never expecting anything back – I've never experienced anything like it before." Likewise, participant A said, "Dave allowed me to totally forget financial and logistics management – what a gift that was. It was not an easy task, but what a trooper. I am so grateful. As well, the group had the elasticity to bring him into the thought processes – which he relished. He's a human resources professional out of West Point – and was always eager to learn." There was unanimity among the group that the project manager had made everyone's lives easier and that he became a participant in the group activities and conversations.

Regarding the foundation representative's participation, opinions were more varied. For example, participant E stated, "There wasn't just some money bags in the sky who gave a grant, but the granting agency had a person who was a regular participant and I think that that was really, really important. And when I say participant, I don't mean spy. I wondered on day one, 'What is this guy's role?' but he was there in soul and the spy paranoia just dissipated. I think it was just a wonderful idea on the part of whoever it was to have him as a regular group member." Participant G was less enthusiastic and stated, "I remember always feeling a little mystified by him – whether he was judging what we were doing – or our audience and if so were we doing ok? So . . . I held him a little at bay."

As was true for other aspects of the RCCRN, a spirit of community and inquiry prevailed, even to the extent that the project manager and funding representative became active and contributing members of the activities and dialogs that took place during the face-to-face meetings. One of the precepts of community-based participatory research is that every person regardless of their role or station in life has something to contribute to the research enterprise. That was no more evident than in the RCCRN. Participant B summarized this poignantly by stating, "I think everybody played a role. . . . Everybody was a part of it. I didn't always know what they were doing, but it didn't really matter to me. They always participated and were interesting and I grew to care about them just as I grew to care about everybody else in the network."

Funding

As mentioned at the beginning of this chapter, funding for the research network was provided by the Fetzer Institute, a working foundation in Kalamazoo, Michigan. The principal investigators (Inui and Frankel) had written a general description of what the research initiative was designed to accomplish but the process and scholarly output of the initiative was framed in terms of "emergent design;" that is, an understanding that the processes and outcomes would be defined by the network and its processes.[9] In essence, funding for the research to be undertaken by the network was in hand before specific topics had been selected. We were interested to know from the perspectives of the participants what effect(s) having funding in hand had on members' experiences and asked, "As you recall, funding for the network and its research activities was already in hand before the first meeting. What difference, if any, did this make in terms of your thinking about research and your willingness to collaborate with others?"

Without exception, network members experienced the availability of research funds as freeing them to think creatively and work on projects that were highly motivating to them. For instance, participant H stated, "I think that you don't get money unless you have somebody taking charge, taking the initiative, writing the proposal, and going forward, You know, having the money delivered on a promise is difficult to achieve. Having the money in hand made a big difference in the way that everybody connected in our network." Participant D agreed and asserted, "Having the money in hand made a huge difference. We all want to sit around and think with like-minded colleagues but without funding it's hard to make that happen." Likewise, participant J said, "In trying to get grants funded you have to tailor your interests to the work of the funder. The RCCRN was closer to what people would ideally like to do which is to work on what you think is important." Echoing this sentiment, participant B opined, "Having the money in hand let us think about what we thought was most important as opposed to what is most likely to get a grant funded. I think it absolutely, completely changed the way in which we thought about the research projects."

In summary, members of the RCCRN expressed the view that having funding for the initiative in hand lent itself to the creativity and productivity of the group, and at least indirectly raised the question of whether the current mechanisms for doing science and discovery are limiting because individual researchers are forced to remain in a straight, narrow box to obtain funding. Being able to reach consensus on topics of interest to group members plus being able to explore new ideas and approaches without having to worry about competing against one another for scarce resources gave the group space and time to develop their ideas and methods to pursue them. As one participant, E, put it, "In the real world of scientific clinical investigators, the Relationship-centered Research Network was our Camelot."

Work Products

At the second meeting of the RCCRN, two processes central to scholarly activities were begun: (1) collaboration on developing a working definition of Relationship-Centered Care that could inform research, education, and practice; and (2) deciding upon a research agenda. The outcome of the first process was a paper authored by Mary Catherine Beach, Thomas Inui and the Relationship-Centered Care Network that appeared in the *Journal of General Internal Medicine*, entitled, "Relationship-Centered Care: A Constructive Reframing."[10] The paper was a synthesis of work done by network members using their own experiences of communication in health care as a guide to which input from the ethics literature was added.

The outcome of the second process was the emergence of four collaborative research teams and four topics for RCC research. These were: "The Role of Relationships in Mediating the Effects of the Hidden Curriculum;" "Organizational Factors Associated with Relationality in Ambulatory Care;" "Understanding the Influences of Race and Ethnicity on Patient–Physician Interactions: Delving Below the Surface;" and "Interpersonal Sensitivity and Emotional Self-Awareness in Medical Students." By group consensus, funding for the projects was divided equally and amounted to approximately $80 000 per team.

For the duration of the initiative (nine meetings, total) the entire network continued to meet face to face; each meeting lasting a day and a half. The goal of these meetings was to further community learning, provide an opportunity for the research groups to work together, and to hear progress reports and engage in conversations that could synergize the projects. During that period of time, network members were also active in presenting their work in posters, abstracts, workshops, podium presentations and plenary talks at national and international meetings. More than a dozen peer-reviewed papers were produced by the four work groups over the course of the nine face-to-face meetings with several appearing as late as 2011, and one published in early 2012. Citations to the work of the network have also been frequent in the literature. Papers from each of the research projects were published in a special issue of the *Journal of General Internal Medicine*, January 2006, entitled "Re-Forming Relationships in Healthcare." This single issue (one of 17 *JGIM* issues in the year 2006) had six of the top 20 articles published in *JGIM* for 2005 to 2006, using full-text downloads as the objective quality criterion. A bibliography of papers, presentations, and other work products appears in Appendix 2. Considered on the basis of a return on investment, one would be hard-pressed to conclude that the addition of community formation as a goal of creating a research network had anything but a positive effect on its productivity, as measured by publication in peer-reviewed journals and other forms of scholarship.

Conclusion

We began this chapter with a question about what would happen if instrumental and interpersonal goals were merged in the context of creating and sustaining a research network. To answer this question we used participants' recollections based on in-depth interviews. More than seven years after the start of the initiative some participants still had vivid recollections of how the first meeting of the network began; others recalled the feeling, if not the details, and almost all remarked on how important the focus on personal relationships, including meeting in members' homes, was in setting the tone for the work that was to come. When compared with the goals of the first and subsequent meetings, there was a direct parallel between the intentions of the leaders of the network to integrate instrumental and interpersonal dimensions in creating the network and participants' recollections.

Likewise, when asked to recall the impact of the setting on the process and outcomes of the work, participants noted that meeting in one another's homes provided a broader and richer picture of the host or hostess as well as blurring the boundary between work and family in a positive way. Once established, the sense of being together in a family-like setting took precedence over physical surroundings, such as meeting in a hotel. As one participant stated explicitly and others reflected a little less directly, the meetings in which participants could show up fully (as hosts or hostesses, family members, spouses, etc.) led to more long-lasting and meaningful relationships and research. The setting for these relationships to develop transcended differences in theoretical and methodological orientation, age, gender, and career stage, all of which could have been divisive, but wound up being a community resource instead.

While the effects of physical environment have been studied in many settings such as classroom design,[11] instrumentation in aviation,[12] and hospital design for patients with dementia,[13] scant attention has been paid to the effect(s) of physical context on developing and sustaining research and research relationships. RCCRN members reported multiple benefits from paying close attention to creating a welcoming physical environment and linking the environment to activities known to stimulate creative thinking, such as checking in at the beginning of meetings and debriefing at their conclusion, and using personal narratives, music, poetry, and the arts to create a balance between right-brain and left-brain functions. Our experience suggests that once having set a precedent of meeting in the relaxed surroundings of someone's home it is possible to achieve something of the same result in a more narrowly proscribed environment like a classroom or hotel meeting room.

In addition to the impact of physical setting on group process, attention was paid to the human environment and the web of relationships that were an important part of the RCCRN. The majority of participants were appreciative of having an external facilitator to create and manage a trustworthy invitational process, although some found the process more engaging and consistent with their personal styles than others. As well, reasons for feeling grateful varied. At least one senior member of the group was grateful for being relieved of a responsibility that they usually took on in a group. Being freed of that responsibility allowed this individual to concentrate on creative work and not having to worry about how others in the group were faring. Others felt that having an external facilitator enabled them to participate and "show up" more fully as members of a research community.

The use of facilitated dialog and small group discussion has been found helpful in medical education,[14,15] faculty development,[16] and organizational culture change.[6] External facilitators are often able to help bring about change by virtue of their perceived neutrality and their ability to mediate difficult or complex conversations. Having an independent facilitator for the RCCRN was pivotal in helping to put the human dimension of research (particularly "relationship-centered research") front and center at the beginning of the initiative and served to establish guiding principles for relating during subsequent meetings. Some of these principles, such as appreciative check-in and debriefs, became ritualized expectations in the group whether the facilitator was present or not. Such ritualized activities were one indication that a self-organizing community of research and scholarship had formed and was functioning. While there had been an intention to create community from the beginning of the initiative, the actual functioning of the network was very much self-organizing and self-sustaining once the intention had been made explicit in the first meeting.[17] So well established was the group's ability to function that when one of the co-leaders of the group had to step aside because of a family illness, her replacement (DGS) was able to step in and was seamlessly integrated by the group into her new role.

Should all research groups have an external facilitator? We would argue that an external facilitator is a wonderful addition to any group but is probably not an absolute necessity and, from our interview data, is not every investigator's preference. More important are issues of mindfulness about group formation, attention to the physical and emotional environment, and invitations and activities designed to optimize creativity. In the case of the RCCRN, use of a facilitator was deliberate, and part of our effort to "detoxify" the competitive culture in which participants were embedded and guide them into a formation process that could result in their "embodying" Relationship-Centered Care phenomena. To our knowledge, these principles have not been applied or studied in any formal way in creating research communities, although doing so would not add a great deal of effort or expense.

Finally, members of the RCCRN were unanimous in voicing their praise for the freedom that having funding in hand before setting out to do research together had many benefits in terms of creativity and opportunity to think collaboratively. It is probably not realistic to think that the conditions under which the RCCRN worked will become commonplace. Nevertheless, there are some lessons from this experiment where research dollars were already in hand that can be applied to competition for scarce resources. First, we heard several voices reflect on the fact that the RCCRN allowed them to work on a project for which they had real passion. Finding ways to maintain and prioritize one's research so that it intersects with one's passion is critical. In a trustworthy environment being able to say to colleagues, whose research may take place in the same general domain, what one is honestly thinking about and committed to can help maintain a healthy balance and stimulate growth and development. Second, being a member of a community of practice can be an antidote to feelings of burnout and discouragement, especially if a project or grant does not get funded or produce expected results. Finally, being free of, or at least discussing what it would be like to be free of, the constraints of "following the money" may add to one's creative energy and willingness to take chances on ideas that one is passionate about but may have limited or no funding available. In the RCCRN, we urged group participants to push beyond the bounds of incremental thinking. Having the money up front, in some real sense, compelled us to take risks and jump conceptually beyond what we knew could be funded by ordinary study section proposals. It's also noteworthy that the group decided to divide the available funding equally, instead of investing it in some other way. The return on this very modest investment in each of the four projects, judging by the number of independent publications, is remarkable.

In the 1950s Michael Balint, a British psychiatrist, began organizing groups of physicians who came together with the sole purpose of talking and sharing stories about what made medicine meaningful for them and what obstacles got in the way of their feeling fulfilled by their chosen profession.[18] One of the consistent themes from the work of Balint, and others who have continued in his tradition, is the value of creating intense interpersonal relationships in small groups as a means of combating burn-out, isolation, and loneliness. Balint, and other organizations such as the American Academy on Communication in Healthcare, have implemented personal awareness groups whose goal is to create a safe space for health-care professionals to engage deeply with others about what is meaningful for them.[19] Our experience of creating community in the Relationship-Centered Research Network suggests that similar processes could be used among individuals and teams of researchers to create a deeper sense of community and commonality than currently seems to exist.

In closing, we note that the predominant view of science in the modern era (from the turn of the 20th century on) is saturated with war metaphors. For example, we "defend" our hypotheses and "attack" the other's position and do so largely without regard for the other's perspective. Research done within this paradigm has been very successful but also runs the risk of stripping away interpersonal relationships as a legitimate source of discovery and creativity in doing science. Despite calls for more collaboration and quicker translation of evidence into practice, which implies more functional ways of relating, the overarching paradigm has not really changed in more than a century.

The RCCRN produced more that was both innovative and of deep value (evidenced by the *JGIM* download statistics, among other things) with far fewer resources than is normally required for such scientific endeavors. What made this work so productive? Perhaps being freed from the practical consideration of having to worry about funding was part of what made the network successful, but there was also something deeper. Over and over in our interviews with network participants we heard comments about how freeing it was to be able to relate to others personally as well as professionally. Some structured ways of interacting such as the use of check-ins was one important (and highly untraditional) way that we created personal engagement; meeting in people's homes rather than institutions was another, as was hiring an independent facilitator. These three ingredients (check-ins to start every conversation, selecting more intimate settings for our discussions, and facilitation) were ways of freeing the group from the ordinary constraints of "doing science." We were able to think more deeply together and we invented things, generated ideas, did work and produced papers with relatively few resources and with ease and joy. Although terms like "ease" and "joy" are not currently part of the dominant lexicon of rigorous scientific inquiry, our experience with the RCCRN raises the intriguing possibility that value is added when research is done by engaging the "whole" person. In the end, perhaps Inui's admonition[2] about the need to educate physicians to engage fully as persons and professionals can fruitfully be extended to the lives of researchers as well. Time will tell.

Acknowledgments

The authors would like to acknowledge The Fetzer Institute of Kalamazoo for their generous support of the Relationship-Centered Research Initiative and to David Sluyter, EdD for his role both as a liaison between Fetzer and the Research Initiative and as an active member in its activities. Both were much appreciated.

Appendix 1: Interview Questions

We are co-authoring a chapter for a book on research in academic health centers and are interested in learning about your experience as a member of the Relationship-Centered Research Initiative. I would like to interview you for about 30 minutes and learn more about what it was like to become part of the network, your experiences during the time that it was active, and any long-term effects participation has had for you.

First, as you think back about the RCCRI do you have any distinct memories or response to having been asked to join the network? If so, can you describe what they were?

● Was it an easy or difficult decision to join? Why?

- Did you have any particular fears or concerns about joining the group?
- How well did you know others in the network and what effect(s) did knowing or not knowing others have on you and your willingness to participate?

Next, I'd like to ask you some questions about the formation of the group and how it compares with other research collaboratives that you have participated in.
- How did you imagine the group process would work?
- Did that turn out to be the case? What happened that you did not expect?
- Overall – did the group process change you over time or feel consistent and steady?
- Please recall the evening of our first gathering as a group. What stands out for you from that meeting? As you think about other research collaboratives that you have participated in was there anything unusual of different that you noticed about the beginning of the initiative?
- Early on we decided to meet in people's homes rather than in institutional settings. What difference(s) if any did the change in venue make for you personally? In terms of group formation?
- As we began the initiative there were many standing relationships and natural subgroups within the network. Please describe a subgroup that you were in at the beginning of the initiative and what happened to that subgroup during the course of our meetings.
- There were a number of strong professional differences (theory, method, funding, etc.) that marked the group. What was your experience of those differences at the beginning of the initiative? How, if at all, did these change over time?
- In addition to the identified researchers in the group we also invited Penny to join us as a network facilitator. In what ways do you think her presence affected the group's formation and functioning? Can you recall a specific moment or time when her presence made a positive difference for you as an individual? For the group? Please tell the story of those times.

Finally, I'd like to ask you some questions about the long-term effect(s) of the initiative on your thinking about research and collaboration.
- Have you belonged to a research collaborative in the past?
- If so, what was that group like (culture, duration, context)? How does the RCC compare?
- If not, were you looking for that kind of experience?
- What impact, if any, do you feel participating in the RCCRN has had on you personally and professionally? In the short run? In the long term?

- As you recall, funding for the network and its research activities was already in hand before the first meeting. What difference, if any, did this make in terms of your thinking about research and your willingness to collaborate with others? At the beginning of the initiative? Now?
- Can you think of a specific incident or experience in which collaboration was enhanced or impeded by the way the network was formed and facilitated?
- Finally, in addition to the researchers and facilitator there were other members of the group including the project manager and a representative from Fetzer. From your perspective what role did they play in your experience of the initiative?
- In retrospect were there aspects of the group process that you would have liked to change in some way?

Are there any comments you'd like to add? Anything I've missed?

Thank you for your time and willingness to participate in this interview.

Appendix 2: Relationship-Centered Care Research Network Publications
••••••••••••••••••••••••

- Beach MC, Inui TS with the Relationship-Center Care Research Network (Frankel R, Hall J, Haidet P, Roter D, Beckman H, Cooper LA, Miller W, Mossbarger D, Safran D, Sluyter D, Stein H, Williamson P). Relationship-centered care: a constructive reframing. *J Gen Intern Med.* 2006; **21**(Suppl. 1): S3–8.
- Blanch DC, Hall JA, Roter DL, Frankel RM. Medical student gender and issues of confidence. *Patient Educ Couns.* 2008; **72**(3): 374–81.
- Blanch DC, Hall JA, Roter DL, Frankel RM. Is it good to express uncertainty to a patient? Correlates and consequences for medical students in a standardized patient visit. *Patient Educ Couns.* 2009; **76**(3): 300–6.
- Blanch-Hartigan D, Hall JA, Roter DL, Frankel RM. Gender bias in patients' perceptions of patient-centered behaviors. *Patient Educ Couns.* 2010; **80**: 315–20.
- Cooper LA, Roter DL, Carson KA, Beach MC, Sabin JA, Greenwald AG, Inui TS. Implicit racial bias among clinicians, communication behaviors, and patient ratings of interpersonal care. *Am J Public Health.* **102**(5): 979–87.
- Cooper LA, Beach MC, Johnson RL, Inui TS. Delving below the surface: understanding how race and ethnicity influence relationships in healthcare. *J Gen Intern Med.* 2006; **21**(Suppl. 1): S21–7.
- Frankel RM, Inui TS. Re-forming relationships in health care: papers from the 9th Bi-Annual Regenstrief Conference. *J Gen Intern Med.* 2006; **21**(Suppl. 1): S1–2.
- Haidet P, Hatem D, Fecile ML, Stein H, Haley HL, Kimmel B, Mossbarger D, Inui T. The role of relationships in the professional formation of physicians: case report and illustration of an elicitation technique. *Patient Educ Couns.* 2008; **72**(3): 382–7.

- Haidet, P, Stein H. The role of the student–teacher relationship in the formation of physicians: the hidden curriculum as process. *J Gen Int Med.* 2006; **21**(Suppl. 1): S16–20.
- Hall JA, Roter DL, Blanch DC, Frankel RM. Observer rated rapport in interactions between medical students and standardized patients. *Patient Educ Couns.* 2009; **3**: 323–7.
- Hall JA, Roter DL, Blanch DC, Frankel RM. Nonverbal sensitivity in medical students: implications for clinical interactions. *J Gen Intern Med.* 2009; **24**(11): 1217–22.
- Roter DL, Frankel RM, Hall JA, Sluyter D. The expression of emotion through nonverbal behavior in medical visits: mechanisms and outcomes. *J Gen Intern Med.* 2006; **21**(Suppl. 1): S28–34.
- Roter DL, Hall JA, Blanch-Hartigan DC, Larson S, Frankel RM. Slicing it thin: new methods for brief sampling analysis using RIAS-coded medical dialogue. *Patient Educ Couns.* 2011; **82**(3): 410–19.
- Safran DG, Miller W, Beckman H. Organizational dimensions of relationship-centered care. Theory, evidence, and practice. *J Gen Intern Med.* 2006; **21**(Suppl. 1): S9–15.

References

1. Sillitoe A. *The Loneliness of the Long-Distance Runner.* London: W.H. Allen; 1959.
2. Inui TS. *A Flag in the Wind: educating for professionalism in medicine.* Washington, DC: Association of American Medical Colleges; 2003.
3. Cresswell JW. *Qualitative Inquiry and Research Design: choosing among five traditions.* Newbury Park, CA: Sage Publications; 1998.
4. Crabtree BF, Miller WLE. *Doing Qualitative Research.* 2nd ed. Thousand Oaks, CA: Sage Publications; 1999.
5. Suchman A, Williamson P, Litzelman D, *et al.* Towards an informal curriculum that teaches professionalism: transforming the social environment of a medical school. *J Gen Intern Med.* 2004; **19**(5): 501–4.
6. Cottingham AH, Suchman AL, Litzelman DK, *et al.* Enhancing the informal curriculum of a medical school: a case study in organizational culture change. *J Gen Intern Med.* 2008; **23**(6): 715–22.
7. Tresolini CP, Pew-Fetzer Task Force. *Health Professions Education and Relationship-centered Care: report of the Pew-Fetzer Task Force on advancing psychosicial education.* San Francisco, CA: Pew Health Commission; 1994.
8. Palmer P. *A Hidden Wholeness: the journey toward an undivided life.* San Francisco: Jossey-Bass; 2004.
9. Schwandt T. *The SAGE Dictionary of Qualitative Research.* 3rd ed. Thousand Oaks, CA: Sage Publications; 2007. p. 79.
10. Beach MC, Inui TS, Relationship-centered Care Research Network. Relationship-centered care: a constructive reframing. *J Gen Intern Med.* 2006; **21**(Suppl. 1): S3–8.
11. Higgens S, Hall E, Wall K, *et al.* *The Impact of School Environments: a literature review.* Newcastle, UK: University of Newcastle; 2005.
12. Alexander AL, Wickens CD, Hardy TJ. Synthetic vision systems: the effects of guidance symbology, display size, and field of view. *Hum Factors.* 2005; **47**(4): 693–707.
13. Day K, Carreon D, Stump C. The therapeutic design of environments for people with dementia: a review of the empirical research. *Gerontologist.* 2000; **40**(4):397–416.
14. Branch WT Jr. Use of critical incident reports in medical education. A perspective. *J Gen Intern Med.* 2005; **20**(11): 1063–7.
15. Branch WT Jr., Frankel R, Gracey CF, *et al.* A good clinician and a caring person: longitudinal faculty development and the enhancement of the human dimensions of care. *Acad Med.* 2009; **84**(1): 117–25.
16. Kumagai AK, White CB, Ross PT, *et al.* The impact of facilitation of small-group discussions

of psychosocial topics in medicine on faculty growth and development. *Acad Med*. 2008; **83**(10): 976–81.

17. Stacey R. *Complexity and Creativity in Organizations*. San Francisco: Berrett-Koehler; 1996.

18. Scheingold L. Balint work in England: lessons for American family medicine. *J Fam Pract*. 1988; **26**(3): 315–20.

19. Kern DE, Wright SM, Carrese JA, *et al.* Personal growth in medical faculty: a qualitative study. *West J Med*. 2001; **175**: 92–8.

9

Successful Aging in Research

Supporting Generativity across Generations

*Bruce M. Psaty and David S. Siscovick**

Bruce Psaty's Story of a Success in Science: Following the Road Less Travelled in Funding Research

I enjoy writing, tinkering with prose, and write well so literary products are often personally satisfying. They come to closure when they are right where I want them. A good example was the CHARGE infrastructure grant. That grant application had no hypotheses. The sole purpose was to provide support to each of the major cohort studies that are contributing data to the CHARGE consortium and to provide coordinating center support for the activities of the consortium as a whole. The CHARGE consortium is an investigator-initiated voluntary federation among cohort studies. There was no funding and no organizational support for the consortium itself. The investigators just decided it would be useful to collaborate, and indeed it has been. They had no support for conference calls or for meetings. Having

---

* **Affiliations:** From the Cardiovascular Health Research Unit, Departments of Medicine (Psaty, Siscovick), Epidemiology (Psaty, Siscovick), and Health Services (Psaty), University of Washington and Group Health Research Institute, Group Health Cooperative, Seattle, Washington (Psaty, Siscovick).

Grants: This research was supported in part by grants HL078888, HL080295, HL085251, HL087652, HL103612, and HL105756 (Psaty) and HL088456, HL088576, HL091244, and HL092111 (Siscovick) from the National Heart, Lung, and Blood Institute. The content is solely the responsibility of the authors and does not necessarily represent the official views of the National Heart, Lung, and Blood Institute or the National Institutes of Health.

worked for many years at coordinating centers, I saw the need and wrote a grant application to provide organizational support in part from the Cardiovascular Health Research Unit, which my colleagues at the University of Washington and I established, and in part from the Collaborative Health Studies Coordinating Center of the University of Washington. This grant application also included an opportunity for what we called "fellowship exchanges," which have been successful to date. The budget included $50,000 per year, $10,000 per student or fellow, to go to another institution and visit. That visit had to be tied to a particular paper that a consortium working group was developing. Principals at the receiving and the sending institution both had to agree to this work and arrangement. There had to be a vision of at least short-term and potentially long-term products of this exchange. With this grant, the consortium members have been able to exchange and support fellows, graduate students, and post-docs among institutions to acquire experience at another institution that they wouldn't have had by remaining at their own institution. The grant received a *perfect* score in peer review at the NHLBI.

David Siscovick's Story of a Success in Science: Persistence Pays Off

The area of sudden cardiac arrest is clearly my passion. It was a challenge to get others to recognize that this is a suitable focus for research. In the Jewish tradition there's this concept of Mazal, commonly translated as "luck or good fortune" that you may have heard about. The Hebrew letters are Mem, Zayin, Lamed. There is a teaching that Mem stands for Makom which is place, the Zayin stands for Zimon which is time and the Lamed stands for Lashone which is speech – you have to be in the right place at the right time and say the right thing to have luck or good fortune. So luck isn't just luck; it's being at the right place at the right time and saying the right thing.

I wanted to collect blood in population-based studies of sudden cardiac arrest so that I could use it to evaluate biomarkers and so I would have the opportunity to store white cell pellets which have DNA in them. Several key collaborators, Len Cobb, Mike Copass and Micky Eisenberg, were supportive of my coming to Seattle and indicated a willingness to work with me to see if we could get the emergency-response system paramedics to draw blood for our studies. Paramedics typically started IVs in Seattle when they attended patients, so the question was whether they could draw blood at the time they were starting the IV or some time later after a resuscitation was completed and the patient was clinically stable. This was for fatal cases as well as non-fatal cases. We also obviously had to get approval from our IRB to do this and because we were not in a position to get informed consent in the emergency medical care setting our IRB worked with us and gave us approval to review paramedic incident reports and to have the paramedics collect samples from individuals in the field, providing those samples to our study. With pilot funding from the Seattle MedicOne Foundation and from the Clinical Nutrition Research Unit, we were able to generate pilot data that enabled us to get an R01. In 1988, NHLBI was scoring applications 100 to 500, from the first percentile to the 100th percentile. My first application was in the 92nd percentile. It was as far away from getting funded as you can imagine. It had no preliminary data, just an idea. The second proposal, the revision was in the 55th percentile. It had preliminary data on dietary assessment using spouse respondents (since 90% of the cases are fatal) and was in the 55th percentile. The second revision, which was allowed in those days, included data from 18 primates in which we measured biomarkers in red blood cell membranes before and after the animals were sacrificed. The pilot data on 18 primates was included in the application, and that application was scored in the 12th percentile and was funded. We subsequently had two competitive renewals to continue our work on biomarkers of fatty acids and sudden death and were funded for over 15 years to do work on dietary intake, fatty acid biomarkers and sudden cardiac arrest. That process of doing research around a focused question but at the same time creating resources for additional questions is what led to our being positioned to do something in the area of genetic associations with sudden death, once the technology for high throughput genomics, such as candidate gene, genome-wide association (GWAS), and exome chip studies were available to study genetic associations in unrelated individuals. As a result of the pilot funding from the MedicOne Foundation and from the CNRU, we have actually had seven R01s over the course of 20 years and have created a resource that's now not only being used by us but is also being used internationally through the collaborative network CHARGE to combine our data from other studies of sudden death, providing data for nearly all of the studies that are looking at determinants of sudden death in the United States and Europe.

Introduction
••••••••••••••••••

Successful aging in biomedical research requires scientific collaboration across generations. Economic support has been provided through National Institutes of Health training grants (T32 awards) and early career development awards (K-awards). However, little attention has been given to social and cultural factors that influence individual and institutional behaviors and promote generativity across generations. For example, the focus on the individual contributor, the competition for novel discoveries, and the emphasis on the promotion of individual careers rather than the health of the scientific community, have resulted in barriers to mentorship, collaboration, and the sharing of research resources. Mentorship of young scientists sharpens research questions, collaboration among young and senior scientists enhances productivity, and the sharing of research resources in physical or virtual laboratories increases the power to examine clinical research questions. In this chapter, we share our efforts to promote generativity across generations and improve the health of the public. We adopted a model that includes mentorship, collaboration, and the development and sharing of resources; the model now has been used successfully in multiple research settings and by multiple groups; and the model has improved the productivity of many scientists and promoted the career development of early- and mid-career researchers. This model has the potential to transform the culture of science for individuals and research institutions, including academic institutions and the NIH.

The year 2011 is the 20th anniversary of the Cardiovascular Health Research Unit (CHRU), a research center we founded and continue to co-direct. After medical school and residency, both of us received research training at the University of Washington's Robert Wood Johnson Clinical Scholars Program under the co-direction of James LoGerfo and Thomas Inui. Independently, our fellowship work focused on cardiovascular disease epidemiology and prevention. By the mid-1980s, both of us had been recruited as faculty to the Departments of Medicine and Epidemiology at the University of Washington. While these recruitments co-located us and provided us with the opportunity to work together, the choice whether or not to do so was entirely ours. Within several years, we both had secured NIH grants. We were aware of successful collaborative models of research that integrated cardiovascular epidemiology and biostatistics. We wanted to build an interdisciplinary program focused on cardiovascular epidemiology and prevention; and, we were fortunate that our mentor, Edward Wagner, who shared our goals and then was the director of the Group Health Cooperative (GHC) Center for Health Studies, allowed us to sublease space from GHC. His support enabled us to conduct research efforts efficiently and to build an interdisciplinary program of research in collaboration with a large HMO. In 1991, the 3000 square feet of space, located on the 13th floor of an office building where the GHC Center for Health Studies occupied floors 14–16 and the Fred Hutchinson Cancer Research Center occupied floors 2–11, had to be built out, staff had to be hired, data collection efforts were just getting under way, and data to write papers were few.

Currently, the CHRU houses nine faculty, 33 scientists and staff, and 11 students, eight of whom are on a Cardiovascular Disease Training Grant (T32) from the National Heart, Lung and Blood Institute. Between 1991 and 2011, the CHRU faculty brought in about $85 million in grants and contracts, all of it from public or non-profit sources. In case-control studies conducted at GHC, we have reviewed more than 48 000 medical records, about half of whom have been eligible for our studies. Since 1995, we have collected and stored blood specimens on more than 10 000 participants. In case-control studies in the community, we have obtained blood specimens on more than 600 cases of early-age at onset myocardial infarction (MI) and 5000 cases of sudden death in the community, as well as control subjects for these studies. Over the years, we have helped to design and conduct major NHLBI-funded cohort studies, including the Cardiovascular Health Study (CHS), the Multi-Ethnic Study of Atherosclerosis (MESA) Study, and the Coronary Artery Risk Development in Young Adults (CARDIA) Study. With the advent of genome-wide association studies (GWAS) and sequencing studies, the CHRU now houses terabytes of genetic data on tens of thousands of subjects from population-based studies, as well as clinical, survey, examination, and biomarker data. Recently, we have helped to foster international collaborations among cohort studies such as the Cohorts for Heart and Aging Research in Genomic Epidemiology (CHARGE). Together, we have published 841 papers and are co-authors on 114.

After establishing ourselves as seasoned investigators, we focused much of our effort and time on developing the careers of young investigators, locally, nationally, and internationally. As we reflect on the history of our research unit and careers, we recognize that we have been fortunate in many ways. The three major themes that emerge are mentoring, collaboration, and the development and sharing of research resources. Below, we provide additional information about the local studies in Seattle, the national collaborations, and the international efforts including research networks and consortia. These studies, which expand in reach and scope over time, provide a framework for developing the main themes that seem to have contributed to the successful aging of the CHRU: mentorship, collaboration, and the sharing of research resources.

A Patchwork of Cardiovascular Case-control Studies at Group Health Cooperative (Bruce)

The traditional design for studies of cardiovascular disease is the cohort study. The Framingham Heart Study (FHS), launched in 1948 and still under way as a family study, is the classic example. Our mentors – Tom Inui, Jim LoGerfo, Ed Wagner, Noel Weiss and Tom Koepsell – were largely non-denominational in terms of both study design and phenotype, although there was perhaps a slight bias toward case-control studies, which were commonly used in studies of cancer etiology by investigators at the Fred Hutchinson Cancer Research Center.

I (BP) would love to tell you that my current activities in drug safety, pharma-coepidemiology, and pharmacogenetics represent the culmination of a life-long plan; but in truth, early on, my own research interests expressed in terms of outcomes and exposures were ill-defined and thus ecumenical. From the start, I nonetheless had a preference for high-quality data. In an early project on anemia at Indiana University, I used the Regenstrief Institute electronic medical record data retrieval system to identify patients who had had a bone marrow test and then went to the laboratory to review the complete reports and bone-marrow slides from selected cases. The electronic records, which are typically administrative files developed and used for purposes other than research, served as pointers, and for the conduct of high-quality studies, additional effort is required to validate events, exposures or covariates.

In 1983, the year before I came to Seattle, Ed Wagner had started the Center for Health Studies (now the Group Health Research Institute) at Group Health Cooperative. He welcomed my work at Group Health and helped facilitate it. At the time, Group Health had administrative records that identified all members, billing records that captured information about discharge diagnoses, and a computerized pharmacy system that captured every outpatient prescription dispensed to all enrollees since 1976.

The electronic files at Group Health were well suited to the conduct of population-based case-control studies. In a study of myocardial infarction, for instance, the diagnostic data could serve as pointers to potential events that could be verified by medical-record review. Cases should represent all the events in a defined population, and controls should be sampled from the same population from which the cases arose. The cancer case-control studies typically used the community cancer registry to identify cases in a geographic area; as a result, to obtain a sample of population-based controls, the cancer epidemiologists often used the complex method of random-digit dialing. At Group Health, the health-maintenance-organization's enrollment files defined the population from which the perfect controls could be sampled easily and inexpensively. The computerized pharmacy database also represented an outstanding source of information about prescription drugs. Patient recall, especially for past use, may not be reliable, and medical records are sometimes incomplete. But patients do not continue to refill prescription medications that are without street value and that they are not using. Our pharmacoepidemiological case-control studies emerged from this confluence of data and mentoring resources.

When I was a third-year medical student, the Hypertension Detection and Follow-up program reported that the treatment of hypertension using a step-care approach that included high-dose diuretics as the first-line agent reduced total mortality. That finding represented powerful prevention. Yet only one randomized trial had compared various first-line agents for the treatment of hypertension in terms of the prevention of major cardiovascular events such as myocardial infarction. My first case-control study at GHC involved an observational study of the comparison between high-dose diuretics and beta-blockers. This early effort in comparative effectiveness research was driven by the epidemiological need to control for confounding by indication. Additionally, we were interested in both the potential benefits and risks of drug therapies. The advantage of the computerized pharmacy records became apparent in a secondary analysis when we showed that non-compliance with beta-blockers was associated with a transient increase in the risk of MI.[1]

The experience gained in conducting this first study created the setting for a series of case-control studies. In the next one, we studied the association of progestin use with MI risk in menopausal women – an idea first suggested by Noel Weiss. A pilot study helped us evaluate methods for identifying stroke cases. The two case groups, MI and stroke, shared a single control group. Soon, many new anti-hypertensive agents were marketed for first-line use in the United States. So we added men with treated hypertension to the study of postmenopausal women, which already included women with treated hypertension.[2] In his studies, David Siscovick was already drawing blood and storing specimens, including DNA, on sudden death cases. We took advantage of his experience and submitted a competing supplement to draw blood on the cases and controls in our GHC studies. With each new project, we took advantage of the existing data, expanded the data-collection efforts to address a new question or set of questions, and thereby continued to create new resources for future work.

Although we were never funded to create new systems at Group Health, we regarded the products of our work as research resources. Other questions could be posed and answered within the available datasets. For instance, Susan Heckbert used the incident MI cases identified in our case-control studies to launch a study of prognosis.[3] Using this framework, she created an inception cohort of subjects assembled at the time of their first MI. Under the influence of Frits Rosendaal, who spent a sabbatical year with us in 1995, we added a case group of venous thrombosis. Subsequently, Nick Smith has continued the work on first events of venous thrombosis[4] and added a study of risk factors for second or recurrent events of venous thrombosis. Recently, Susan Heckbert added a case group of patients with atrial fibrillation. Although the control group has evolved over time to accommodate changes in the study questions, a single control group has nonetheless served for all four outcomes: myocardial infarction, stroke, venous thrombosis, and atrial fibrillation.

These related studies have always been treated as a shared resource among collaborating investigators (primarily Heckbert, Smith, and Psaty but also Siscovick and Sotoodehnia). Forms and methods developed in one setting have been adopted or adapted for use in another setting. New activities related to data collection, data entry, and the processing and storage of blood specimens take advantage of previous experience. For instance, once a program has been developed to assess the use of a medication or a class of medications for one project, that program has generally become the local standard, which we have shared not only within the CHRU but also with GHC investigators. The team approach to the conduct of these studies encourages all investigators to partici-pate, contribute, and benefit from the research resources. The research system does not depend on any one person, and so can proceed seamlessly even during travel, vacations, and family emergencies.

Aware that we are benefiting from the resources made available by Group Health, we have contributed our share of service work to the Cooperative, not only in the form of service on committees, but also in terms of enhancing the data systems. At one point, we developed methods for matching the ever-enrolled membership file at Group Health to the Washington State death records for our studies, and we provided the product of the matching effort to GHC programmers for their use on an annual basis for all investigators. Under the leadership of one of our trainees, Gina Schellenbaum Lavasi, we collaborated with GHC investiga-tors to create a geographical information systems (GIS) dataset that was used to examine the built environment, walkability, and incident myocardial infarction.

Case-control Studies of Sudden Cardiac Arrest (SCA)
Death in the Community (David)

I (DS) conducted a population-based case-control study of exercise and SCA in Seattle and King County as a Robert Wood Johnson Clinical Scholar at the UW (1979–81). The work was supported by my first R01 award from NIH; and the study helped to clarify the risks and benefits of exercise as they relate to sudden cardiac arrest.[5,6] While my mentors had advised against doing a large project that required funding, I was both naïve and passionate about the prevention of SCA. For these reasons, I went with my heart and – with the support of my mentors – generated the funding and data to address several novel questions with clinical and public health implications. This early success, spanning five years and two institutions, was critical to what followed.

In the spring of 1981, there still was a nation-wide recession, a budget deficit in most states, and a hiring freeze at the University of Washington. While Tom Inui, then General Internal Medicine Unit Chief at the Seattle VA Medical Center, had planned (before the recession) to keep me as part of his team at Washington, I was "traded" late that spring of 1981 to his colleagues (former Carnegie Commonwealth Clinical Scholars) and friends at the University of North Carolina, Chapel Hill, Robert and Suzanne Fletcher, the new co-heads of the UNC Division of General Internal Medicine, for future considerations. The Fletchers were ideal mentors for an academic general internist-cardiovascular epidemiologist. Within the first five years at Carolina, I had published two of my first three papers in *JAMA* and the *NEJM*, and I was awarded both a Teacher and Research Scholar Award from the American College of Physicians and an NHLBI Preventive Cardiology Academic Award. The recession ended in 1983–4, and Tom Inui became the head of a new Division of General Internal Medicine at the University of Washington in 1985. Tom believed in the Noah's Ark story, two by two, and he and Noel Weiss (Epidemiology) recruited me back to the UW in 1987 as the second young cardiovascular clinical epidemiologist. As a general internist-epidemiologist, I came cheap: no need for a package with wet laboratory, space for a research group, start-up funding, and so forth. In part because of the attention in the media to my research on the risks and benefits of exercise related to sudden cardiac arrest, the deans of both the School of Medicine, Stuart Bondurant, and the School of Public Health, Michelle Ibrahim, met with me to determine if a counter-offer would convince me to remain in Chapel Hill. Since my scientific interest in sudden cardiac arrest and social preferences motivated, at least in part, the decision and since I had been promoted early with tenure at

UNC, I wasn't looking for a package (offer) that I could not refuse from the UW or trying to get something tangible (money, space, personnel) from UNC. In the end, mentors, resources for research, the potential for interdisciplinary collaboration around my passion, and the opportunity to be entrepreneurial trumped job security and the potential to be a gentleman professor. It was hard leaving the Fletchers, after all that they taught me and the personal effort they had taken to launch my career. It also was hard leaving Al Tyroler, who had been my mentor in cardiovascular epidemiology at UNC. Al taught me the virtues of being a "POP," a plain old professor. It was clear to both the Fletchers and Al Tyroler that my heart was in Seattle.

So after six productive years in Chapel Hill, I returned to Seattle, in part, to re-establish a research program focused on the determinants of SCA. With the support of Drs. Leonard Cobb, Michael Copass, and Mickey Eisenberg and the Emergency Medical Systems (EMS) of Seattle and King County (Washington), I was able to have the paramedics collect blood samples in the field for both biomarker and subsequently genetic studies related to incident SCA in the community. With pilot funding from the Seattle Medic One Foundation and the UW Clinical Nutrition Research Unit, I was able to obtain preliminary data on dietary intake of seafood and biomarkers of long-chain n-3 polyunsaturated fatty acid intake that led to an R01 award from NHLBI, an award that was competitively renewed on two occasions.[7] Each of these awards focused on questions related to dietary and/or cell-membrane polyunsaturated fatty acids and the risk of SCA in the community.

Based in part upon the pharmacoepidemiological work of Bruce in the early GHC case-control studies (described earlier in this chapter), I succeeded in obtaining funding from NHLBI to link the EMS datasets from Seattle and King County (Washington) with the GHC enrollment files to examine the risk of SCA associated with anti-hypertensive therapies and the risk associated with other medications that had the potential for proarrhythmia, drug-induced SCA. These studies used a case-control design, used the computerized pharmacy databases to assess current drug therapies, and reviewed ambulatory care records from Group Health for information on risk factors, medical conditions, and indications for medications.

For 20 years, I collected blood samples from SCA cases and controls in our studies of fatty acids. Recognizing that genetic variation may contribute to these events, I saved the white cell pellets, so we could extract DNA later for genetic studies. Taking advantage of the resources of what is now called the Cardiac Arrest Blood Study (CABS) and advances in high throughput genome science, my colleagues, Nona Sotoodehnia, Tom Rea, and Rozenn Lemaitre, and I were able to obtain four R01s to examine genetic associations with SCA risk and outcomes, using both candidate gene and GWAS approaches. The CABS study was converted into the CABS-Repository (CABS-R), which includes EMS care, clinical data from prior and index hospitalizations, blood samples (aliquots of plasma, WBCs (DNA), and RBCs), results of genetic studies, biomarkers, and information on the built environment. The intent is to create an ongoing national resource to examine the determinants and cardiovascular and neurological outcomes of SCA in the community.

National Efforts in NHLBI-funded Cohort Studies (Bruce)

Soon after I (BP) joined the faculty in 1986, the NHLBI released a request for a proposal for a large cohort study of older adults. The NHLBI had already initiated the new cohort studies of young adults and of middle-aged adults, the Coronary Artery Risk Development in Young Adults (CARDIA) Study and the Atherosclerosis Risk in Communities (ARIC) Study. What was to become called the Cardiovascular Health Study (CHS) would study the determinants and progression of both clinical and subclinical disease in adults aged 65 years or older. The request for proposals included field centers to recruit subjects, a central laboratory, reading centers for the major elements of the subclinical disease examination, such as echocardiography, and a statistical coordinating center. At the University of Washington, Dick Kronmal, who had experience at the coordinating center of the Coronary Artery Surgery Study (CASS), invited Pat Wahl, a senior biostatistician, and me as the local, if new, cardiovascular epidemiologist to work with him on the biostatistical coordinating center proposal and, when the contract was awarded, on the CHS project itself.

By the time that the contract was funded, David had joined the faculty. David had experienced the collaborative model of epidemiologists including Herman (Al) Tyroler and Gerardo Heiss who worked with biostatisticians such as Jim Grizzle, O. Dale Williams, Ed Davis, Woody Chambless, and others at UNC Chapel Hill. Over time, the new collaboration that evolved between the biostatisticians and the epidemiologists at the UW as a result of the CHS also was extraordinary. We brought clinical experience and epidemiological training. Dick and Pat brought experience in coordinating center management and biostatistics. Later we would also collaborate on the MESA Coordinating Center.

Collaborative studies, I now realize, have their cultures or personalities. In retrospect, we were especially fortunate in CHS. Senior epidemiologists such as Curt Furberg and Lewis Kuller provided experienced leadership characterized by scientific excellence. Nemat Borhani, together with young, enthusiastic, and thoughtful principal investigators such as Linda Fried, Greg Burke, and Russ Tracy, provoked, produced, and participated in energetic discussions. Dick Kronmal trained us all to think about the CHS Coordinating Center as a service unit dedicated to the conduct of the study and the advancement of its aims. Although Dick has specific and fixed beliefs about selected analytic issues, his dedication to high-quality science and service meant that the coordinating center faculty and staff took responsibility for all sorts of problems, engaged them, and worked to solve them. This approach seemed to influence the behavior of the other principal investigators and scientists, who in general actively sought to contribute in constructive ways.

At the University of Washington, David and I were largely without mentors in cardiovascular disease epidemiology. In the setting of CHS, Lew Kuller at Pittsburgh and Curt Furberg at Wake Forest became our mentors. In addition to the routine interactions for the conduct of the study, they also discussed other ideas, methods, and projects with us; they tirelessly reviewed and commented on papers and drafts of grant proposals; and although we were not part of their institutions, they generously gave their time and energies to the advancement of our careers.

With experts in aging and cardiovascular disease, the CHS was an exciting place to work. Greg Burke, Anne Newman, and Linda Fried brought new ideas such as frailty to the project. Teri Manolio, the NHLBI project officer, managed to garner support for serial magnetic brain imaging studies of the participants. Russ Tracy brought extensive experience in laboratory assay and basic science to the group. He led or contributed to some of the earliest studies of C-reactive protein. Over the years, CHS investigators have published more than 750 papers.

The ethos and culture that developed early in CHS influenced later developments in the scientific organization of the study. In October 2001, David Siscovick and Anne Newman organized the CHS Renal Working Group, which included junior investigators from a number of CHS and non-CHS institutions. This multicenter collaboration was initiated to coordinate epidemiologic research into the interrelationships of kidney impairment and cardiovascular disease. David and Anne led monthly teleconference calls, helped the new investigators understand the design of and data in CHS, helped them draft paper proposals, write manuscripts, and develop grant proposals to fund ancillary studies with new measures of renal function in CHS. The approach was almost biblical: by sharing the CHS data and making it widely available to other investigators, the scientists of CHS received in return the expertise, energy, and enthusiasm of a whole generation of new investigators. The formal working group model is a late manifestation of the generous mentorship that many of us had received not only from Drs. Inui, LoGerfo, Wagner, Weiss, and Koepsell but also from Drs. Kronmal, Wahl, Furberg, Kuller, and others in the early years of CHS. The primary organizing structure is the clinical research (intellectual) content area within a study rather than one's own research unit, department, school or academic institution. In short, the working group model established virtual interdisciplinary laboratories populated both by a few senior mentors and by eager, well-trained, young investigators who had promise and prospects for success but were in need of mentorship, collaboration, and data resources.

The CHS *Renal Working Group*, which has served as the model for other Working Groups in CHS, currently includes 14 investigators with diverse training in nephrology, general internal medicine, cardiovascular epidemiology, and biostatistics who represent eight institutions. This productive collaboration has published 48 papers; and the young investigators have successfully competed for three R01 awards (NHLBI – two; NIA – one), two awards from the American Heart Association, and several faculty development awards. Recent publications from the CHS Renal Working Group have defined the strong associations of cystatin C, a novel biomarker of kidney function, with atherosclerotic cardiovascular disease, heart failure, and mortality.[8] The idea of forming a CHS *Vascular Disease of the Brain Working Group* to address neurological issues gained momentum in 2005. Other active working groups include *Aging Working Group, Heart Failure Working Group*, and the *Diabetes Working Group*. In 2009, the Diabetes Working Group received funding from an NIH grant proposal, led by five new (non-CHS) investigators serving as multiple PIs, to investigate the determinants and consequences of abnormal glucose regulation in older adults. The funding was at the level of a program project grant; and, NHLBI had to provide prior approval for submission of the application. At the time, the PIs were all junior faculty from five different institutions (Beth Israel-Deaconess Hospital (Harvard), Brigham and Women's Hospital (Harvard), Cornell, Johns Hopkins; and the University of California, San Diego); none was from the UW; and none had previously obtained an R01 award from NIH.

Once cohort studies are under way, they take on a life of their own and are difficult to stop. By the early 2000s, the NHLBI was seeking ways to reduce the funding that went to the cohort studies that had started in the 1980s. CHS was selected for de-funding. The investigators were enthusiastic and committed to the study. Eager to keep CHS alive, they were willing to work to maintain funding. With the assistance and encouragement of the Steering Committee, several of the formerly young investigators (Psaty, Burke, and Tracy) developed a "Future of CHS Proposal." In it, we proposed to keep the study running; requested a small amount of core contract funding for the Coordinating Center and the Laboratory; planned to continue key elements of the study, such as events identification and adjudication, running with grant funding from ancillary studies; and promised to enhance access to the publicly funded CHS data as we had started to do in the Renal Working Group. With the assistance of a supportive project officer, Jeannie Olson, the Future of CHS contract was secured.

Anne Newman's ancillary study called "All Stars" provided support for another examination of CHS participants, and this work became a major focus of the Aging Working Group. In this setting, Bruce wrote a grant that received a perfect score of 100 (then on the 100 to 500 scale). The CHS events grant had not a single hypothesis. The entire effort was a service grant to continue data collection on events in CHS participants. Each ongoing and new CHS ancillary study, we argued, would not be well positioned to collect its own events data across multiple sites and share those data with other ancillary studies. Yet a single events grant located in the CHS Coordinating Center and working with the Field Center investigators who had been collecting events data since 1989 would enable multiple old and new ancillary studies to evaluate associations with a variety of clinical events in older adults. Although the grant was well writ-ten and merited a good score, the perfect score of 100 seemed to be a political statement by the study section to the NHLBI that the decision to stop CHS may perhaps have lacked some wisdom. The message received by the NHLBI has sometimes seemed to be that because CHS was able to secure funding from an R01 mechanism, other cohort studies can be de-funded and they should use the same approach that CHS did.

One of the elements of the Future of CHS proposal was the New Investigator Workshop developed by David. As exemplified by the Renal Working Group, the ethos in CHS has favored data sharing: in this way, CHS was able to involve bright new investigators, improve the science, and enhance the productivity of the study. Additionally, mentorship by senior investigators provided the new investigators with knowledge about the study's history, structure, design, and data so that high-quality analyses could be produced efficiently. The workshop model, which targeted new investigators, was intended to expand that effort.

The first workshop was held in March 2005 and the second in May 2007.

They were designed to achieve the four objectives: (1) to facilitate the use of existing CHS resources; (2) to aid in the development of data elements new to CHS; (3) to identify mentored research opportunities; and (4) to identify emerging scientists who can help to lead CHS in the future. David reviewed the abstracts from K-awardees in research areas relevant to CHS, cardiovascular and aging research. He identified those with research interests and skills relevant to the aims of CHS. Approximately 50 new investigators were invited to attend the workshops, with the NIH covering the costs of participation. About 40 new investigators from about 20 different (non-CHS) academic centers accepted the invitation and participated in one or both workshops. At each workshop, we sought to promote the active, effective, and efficient involvement of the new investigators in CHS. Through a series of presentations and materials, the new investigators were introduced to the research opportunities provided by CHS. They had an opportunity to interact with CHS investigators and CHS Coordinating Center staff. The workshops were pitched as a beginning of a collaborative effort with CHS. A major feature of both workshops was small group sessions focused on unique opportunities to address clinical research questions. Importantly, the small group sessions at the workshops formed the nidus for the creation or expansion of CHS working groups.

The new CHS investigators participated in working groups related to their research interests. Working groups formed at the workshops, such as the *Vascular Disease of the Brain Working Group*, have continued to meet on a regular basis and provide opportunities for the advancement of the careers of new investigators. For some of the new CHS investigators, the workshop follow-up with the working group model provided mentorship, collaboration, and data resources not present at their local institutions. The CHS New Investigator Workshops have been so successful that the NHLBI has adopted this model for involving new investigators in other cohorts, as reflected by the summer 2008 session, which focused on CARDIA, MESA, and Framingham and the summer 2010 session, which focused on the Atherosclerosis Risk in Communities (ARIC) Study and the Women's Health Initiative (WHI).

As of March 31, 2011, CHS had published 737 manuscripts with another 23 in press or accepted. During the early years of the projects, almost all the papers were published by CHS investigators. (For ease of reference, we use the term "CHS investigator" to refer to scientists who received funding from the CHS contract and the term "CHS collaborator" to refer to non-CHS investigators who actively contribute to the study by writing papers and grant applications through the ancillary study mechanisms.) In the late 1990s, CHS collaborators began to contribute importantly to the publications. During the 2000s, CHS investigators published as first authors an average of about 10 papers per year; but the number of papers published by CHS collaborators increased from about 10–15 per year in 2000–1 up to more than 75 in the year 2011 (*see* Figure 9.1). Grants submitted for ancillary studies in CHS show a similar pattern. As of March 31, 2011, CHS investigators held 27 active grants or ancillary studies, and collaborators held 61 active grants or ancillary studies. Thanks to CHS mentors and young scientists willing to collaborate with us, the CHS continues today with modest core support from the NHLBI and major support coming from grant applications written by many investigators from across the country. By late 2011, three of the (formerly) young scientists have become co-chairs of CHS Working Groups and members of the CHS Steering Committee; and another young scientist serves on the CHS Publications Committee.

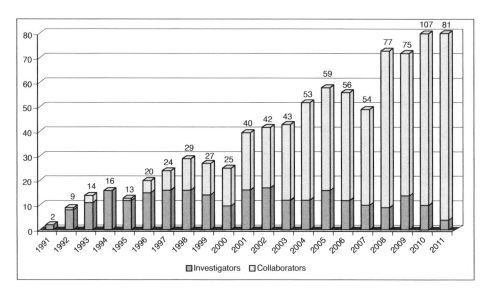

FIGURE 9.1 Annual Number of CHS Manuscripts Published 1991–2011 *(n=866)*

International Efforts: Leiden, Leducq, Jerusalem, and CHARGE (David and Bruce)

In 1995, Frits Rosendaal from Leiden University spent a sabbatical year with us in Seattle. At the time, Frits was a rising star in the field of thrombosis and hemostasis, and he had an interest in oral contraceptives, genes, and venous thrombosis. David and Steve Schwartz had collected DNA in a study of oral contraceptives and incident MI and stroke in premenopausal women in Western Washington, and Frits enabled us to examine the impact of factor V Leiden and a common prothrombin gene variant on MI and stroke in our population-based studies. This visit was the beginning of a number of fruitful collaborations. Under the influence of Frits, Bruce wrote a grant to evaluate potential drug-gene interactions between postmenopausal hormone therapy in women and the factor V Leiden and the prothrombin G20210A variants, associated with clotting risk. The PCR-gel assays were done in Frits' laboratory in Leiden at a cost of $15 per genetic variant. Nowadays, a genome-wide array with a million single-nucleotide polymorphisms costs a few hundred dollars.

The advent of the Internet and electronic mail also facilitated international collaborations. In the early 2000s, Frits and Ted Bovill from the University of Vermont collaborated on a proposal to the Leducq Foundation to create the Leducq International Network Against Thrombosis (LINAT), which included six sites, three in Europe and three in the United States. This study of thrombosis brought together investigators who were well funded and who had diverse and complementary expertise that ranged from population science and biostatistics to mouse models and basic science. The twice-yearly meetings sought to feature the work of young investigators. One of the LINAT project goals was "to promote the exchange of graduate students and post-doctoral fellows . . . so that a network-training program – a virtual graduate school – takes full advantage of the skills and resources at the various sites" (www.med.uvm.edu/pathology/HP-DEPT. ASP?SiteAreaID=728). In the LINAT program, exchanges were an exceptionally effective method of providing students with new experiences not available at their home institutions. The project supported the travel and lodging expenses for young investigators from one site to spend 1–4 months at another site. The exchange had to advance a particular LINAT project that involved collaboration between the two sites. For instance, junior investigators who were training in epidemiology at the University of Washington went to Vermont and Amsterdam to conduct laboratory assays as part of their dissertation efforts.

In 2005, David and Yechiel Friedlander, a genetic epidemiologist from Hebrew University/Hadassah Medical Center (Jerusalem, Israel) were funded to examine whether common genetic variation accounted for the association of maternal pre-pregnancy obesity on cardio-metabolic risk in offspring, using unique data from the Jerusalem Perinatal Study, a historical birth cohort, the recruitment and examination of maternal-adult offspring dyads 30–35 years after birth, and genotyping of candidate gene potentially related to intra-uterine growth and adult cardio-metabolic risk. The NIH support promoted an existing international interdisciplinary collaboration; resulted in an opportunity to add genetic and follow-up data to an existing research resource; offered multiple opportunities for young investigators to address a range of questions related to the developmental (fetal) origins of cardio-metabolic health in offspring; and expanded the mentorship pool for young investigators, both trainees and junior faculty, from the CHRU and Jerusalem. Faculty and post-docs from Jerusalem have worked with CHRU-based research resources; and David has mentored doctoral and post-doctoral students at Hebrew University. The young investigators working on the analysis and reporting of data from the study are likely to make important contributions to our understanding of the determinants of the developmental origins of health and disease.

One of the ancillary studies that helped to provide ongoing support for CHS was a response to a request for applications from the NHBLI for populations to conduct genome-wide association studies (GWAS). As a result, more than 300 000 single-nucleotide polymorphisms were genotyped in about 4000 participants who were free of clinical cardiovascular disease at baseline. The primary aim of the grant was to identify genetic variants associated with the risk of myocardial, stroke, and heart failure although we also recognized the potential to evaluate genetic associations with a large number of other high-quality phenotypes available in a longitudinal study with multiple and repeated measures of risk factors, biomarkers, and measures of subclinical disease.

CHS was one of 14 projects funded to conduct GWAS analyses in the STAMPEED consortium (www.public.nhlbi.gov/GeneticsGenomics/home.stampeed.aspx). Most studies funded by STAMPEED had adequate sample sizes to detect relative risks between about 1.7 and 2.0. By the time that the genotype data were available, however, publications from some of the early GWAS efforts suggested that the effect sizes would be quite modest, median relative risks of about 1.2 to 1.3. For these relative risks, the sample size in CHS, like most every other study, was inadequate. The conduct of high-quality science with valid and reproducible findings would require large sample sizes.

The requirements for large sample sizes and the importance of replication have served as powerful incentives for scientific collaboration. In the late 2000s, GWAS consortia were typically organized around a particular phenotype such as glucose, lipids, or some form of cancer. The primary innovation provided by the CHARGE consortium, formed in February 2008, is the use of the cohort design as the organizing principle. The initial design of the CHARGE Consortium included five prospective aging and cardiovascular cohort studies that first had completed GWAS data from the United States and Europe: Age, Gene/

Environment Susceptibility (AGES) Study, ARIC, CHS, FHS and the Rotterdam Study. Subsequently, other studies such as MESA and CARDIA have joined.

The CHARGE Consortium is an example of an investigator-initiated consortium. CHARGE was formed to facilitate GWAS prospectively planned meta-analyses and replication opportunities among multiple large and well-phenotyped cohort studies.[9] This collaboration, which takes advantage of the hundreds of millions of dollars invested in these cohort studies, is a unique resource for the collaborative investigation of the genetic determinants of multiple phenotypes – risk factors, measures of subclinical disease, and clinical events that were collected in a standardized and comparable fashion. The sharing of results, not individual level data, has facilitated the collaboration and avoided potential IRB concerns about individual-level data sharing. Indeed, the level of collaboration achieved by the CHARGE cohorts is unprecedented.

The CHARGE consortium represents an unfunded voluntary federation of large, complex studies. The organizational structure comprises a Research Steering Committee (RSC), an Analysis Committee, a Genotyping Committee, and approximately 30 phenotype-specific Working Groups. The RSC serves as an administrative executive committee, with shared leadership from each of the five cohorts. The main scientific work in CHARGE takes place in the phenotype-specific Working Groups, which have responsibility for developing and executing the scientific plans. CHARGE adopted both the CHS working group model and its focus on young investigators. The working group model is an effective training ground for students, fellows, and young investigators. With the assistance and guidance of others, the young investigators then have a chance to take a lead as a study representative on a subsequent paper. Many of the young investigators, serving as effective "champions" for their manuscripts, have moved them forward with great energy and enthusiasm. Working groups have tended to reward this collaborative behavior.

In accordance with the original CHARGE principles (http://depts.washington. edu/chargeco/wiki/Main_Page), senior investigators at all sites have made special efforts to include students, fellows, and junior investigators and provide them with the opportunities and the mentoring required for them to serve as leaders of manuscripts about their phenotypes of primary interest. All CHARGE papers have junior investigators among the set of investigators, typically one from each study, who are identified as contributing equally as first authors to the manuscript. The effort to bring these complex papers to fruition often requires a champion, and in the setting of the working-group model, junior investigators have frequently served as effective champions and received mentorship from senior investigators from a variety of sites. To date, CHARGE has more than 75 major GWAS publications, many of them in major journals such as *Nature*, *Nature Genetics*, *New England Journal of Medicine*, and *JAMA*; and perhaps the best measure of its success, about half of the first-first authors of CHARGE meta-analysis papers have been doctoral students, post-doctoral fellows, or junior investigators. A recent grant now supports LINAT-like exchanges for young investigators in CHARGE.

It is important to acknowledge a new kind of mentoring as well. A descriptive though perhaps awkward term for it is "reverse mentoring." In the setting of these large complex projects, young investigators have often acquired skills and expertise in computer systems, analysis techniques, bioinformatics, and the display of complex results – key elements of the current scientific investigations and ones that old-time mentors could not have brought to the consortium.

The large-scale collaborations bring their challenges. The research efforts are far more complex than our early "mom-and-pop" case control studies at Group Health. The work in coordination across multiple complex cohort studies is substantial, and so is the burden of administering multiple subcontracts in funded collaborative projects. To be successful, the consortium members need to abide by a set of principles that include courtesy and transparency. Many consortia, including CHARGE, have developed explicit criteria for participation and data sharing (http://depts.washington.edu/chargeco/wiki/Main_Page). The right of first refusal is, for instance, a principle of courtesy that acknowledges an investigator's known interest in an area, exposure, or phenotype. Letting that person know about an emerging plan and involving him or her in the new work are important for maintaining cohesion and avoiding unnecessary and unproductive controversy. Despite these efforts, some investigators or groups occasionally ignore the rules and conventions. Fortunately, these occurrences are rare, and the exclusion of those who intentionally violate the stated policies and practices required to succeed as a consortium from future collaborations generally leaves them little opportunity for repeat offenses.

CHRU and CHS: Alternatives to Academic Darwinism

In the traditional academic model, physician-investigators are expected to be triple threats – outstanding clinicians, teachers, and researchers. Observations made in the clinical care setting lead to research questions. Advances in basic, clinical, and population science impact the teaching of medicine. While the motivations to pursue a career in research vary, young physician-investigators seek to develop a career in academic medicine and transition from being a "dependent" to an "independent" investigator. Success is measured by the number of funded R01 grants from the National Institutes of Health and the number of first authored publications, especially in high-impact journals. With successful aging, the young investigator transitions to (1) lead a research laboratory (program) at their institution that contributes importantly to the scientific basis of medicine, and (2) the training of post-doctoral research fellows and/or graduate students who then achieve successful academic careers. Competition among investigators within laboratories, institutions, and fields of investigation is considered usual and customary. Even mentors and trainees compete. As in any competitive endeavor, the expectation is that some young investigators will succeed and some will fail; and the fittest young investigators are more likely to survive. The focus is on the success of the individual investigator: the effort is to allocate credit for discoveries to specific individuals. Tenure, where it still exists, is given to individuals based upon their academic record of "independent" research. Contributions to multi-investigator collaborations are given less value than work conducted in a particular laboratory. This traditional, individual contributor approach has been maintained at many academic institutions and at the National Institutes of Health. The negative consequences of this "independent" investigator model on both advances in biomedical science and generativity across the generations have received little attention.

At the University of Washington, we were fortunate to train in the Robert Wood Johnson Foundation Clinical Scholars Program, co-directed by Tom Inui and Jim Logerfo. The Program sought to promote the career development of young physician-scholars, who through training outside of traditional medicine would have the knowledge and skills to be agents of change in medicine. Clinical epidemiology, much like clinical pharmacology, was not a powerhouse in traditional departments of medicine. But with the encouragement of wise senior mentors, we both were selected and chose to pursue clinical scholar training. As with other successful post-doctoral fellowships, the opportunity set us both up for our initial academic appointments and enhanced our likelihood of success in developing successful research careers and promoting generativity across the generations.

Both of us came to Seattle to follow our various passions. While the University of Washington remains a strong traditional biomedical research institution, the research and training culture at the University of Washington has long encouraged innovation and entrepreneurship. There are few barriers across laboratories, divisions, departments, schools, and institutions. Interdisciplinary research has long been valued in this setting. While the university has provided little financial support for our operations, the administrative support provided on several occasions by chairs and deans during the publication of high-profile drug-safety papers was outstanding, encouraging, and enabling. Perhaps fortunately, the area of cardiovascular disease epidemiology and prevention at the University of Washington in the 1980s was completely unfettered by existing institutes, centers, and senior investigators. This freedom from a received tradition in our field allowed us to experiment and to evolve, influenced not only by local mentors without content expertise but also by national mentors with content expertise. The research culture that we developed and promote at the CHRU reflects our own experiences with mentorship, collaboration and the sharing of research resources.

We and others have created virtual (multi-institutional) laboratories in our field that promote collaboration among young investigators, access to data resources, and mentorship from senior investigators. Intentionally, this approach is not centered on one investigator and institution. To some extent, this path is against the traditional grain of academic institutions, as it frequently involves promoting careers of new investigators and even encouraging the development of centers of excellence at other institutions. There are risks: young investigators who follow this path may lack advocates within their institutions among senior faculty; and the contributions of young investigators to multi-authored papers may not be clear, even when they are the first or last author. To be adopted broadly, senior investigators will need to embrace the role of mentorship for those not based in their laboratories, and they will need to enthusiastically collaborate and share resources broadly with the next generation of investigators, both within and outside their institutions. In this model, mentors have the unique opportunity to help shape the research agenda and approach of young investigators interested in a particular content area, but the research agenda and activity of the mentor may need to be modified to accommodate this new role.

The leaders of research institutions, including both academic centers and NIH, will also need to change the research culture and provide appropriate academic rewards, such as appointments, promotions, tenure, and election to distinguished academic research societies, for those who demonstrate excellence in interdependent collaborative research that promotes generativity across the generations and the health of the public. While changing the culture of institutions and the traditional "independent" investigator mindset of some senior faculty is likely to be difficult, we have reasons to be optimistic that this will happen over time. There is mounting evidence of the success of this approach:

the cohort of investigators who benefited from this model now includes mid-career and senior investigators who have become leaders in their scientific fields; and they are now using the principles of mentorship, collaboration, and access to datasets to train their young investigators. Additionally, the NHLBI recently released a novel initiative for funding: it requested proposals for the development of working groups related to heart failure, diabetes mellitus, renal disease, obesity, nutrition, and physical activity, modeled after those in the CHS, to enhance the productivity of another large cohort study, the Jackson Heart Study (JHS). As noted earlier, the NHLBI also has a commitment to the training of the next generation of scientists; and it sees this initiative as an opportunity to promote the research capacity of investigators and institutions with a commitment to minority cardiovascular health. This model has relied on fairly high levels of grant funding from the NIH, and if the paylines fall with a long downturn in the economy, the ability to sustain mentors and young investigators alike may be jeopardized. We suggest that the availability of a funding stream to support the adoption of this non-traditional model will lead to high-impact, high-quality, translational science that promotes the health of the public and generativity across the generations.

Acknowledgment

Thanks to Erika Enright for providing information and the figure on CHS publications through December 31, 2011.

References

1. Psaty BM, Koepsell TD, Wagner EH, et al. The relative risk of incident coronary heart disease associated with recently stopping the use of beta-blockers. JAMA. 1990; **263**(12): 1653–7.
2. Psaty BM, Heckbert SR, Koepsell TD, et al. The risk of myocardial infarction associated with antihypertensive drug therapies. JAMA. 1995; **274**(8): 620–5.
3. Heckbert SR, Kaplan RC, Weiss NS, et al. Risk of recurrent coronary events in relation to use and recent initiation of postmenopausal hormone therapy. Arch Intern Med. 2001; **161**(14): 1709–13.
4. Smith NL, Heckbert SR, Lemaitre RN, et al. Esterified estrogens and conjugated equine estrogens and the risk of venous thrombosis. JAMA. 2004; **292**(13): 1581–7.
5. Siscovick DS, Weiss NS, Fletcher RH, et al. The incidence of primary cardiac arrest during vigorous exercise. N Engl J Med. 1984; **311**(14): 874–7.
6. Siscovick DS, Weiss NS, Hallstrom AP, et al. Physical activity and primary cardiac arrest. JAMA. 1982; **248**(23): 3113–17.
7. Siscovick DS, Raghunathan TE, King I, et al. Dietary intake and cell membrane levels of

long-chain n-3 polyunsaturated fatty acids and the risk of primary cardiac arrest. *JAMA*. 1995; **274**(17): 1363–7.

8. Shlipak MG, Sarnak MJ, Katz R, *et al*. Cystatin C and the risk of death and cardiovascular events among elderly persons. *N Engl J Med*. 2005; **352**(20): 2049–60.

9. Psaty BM, O'Donnell CJ, Gudnason V, *et al*. Cohorts for Heart and Aging Research in Genomic Epidemiology (CHARGE) Consortium: design of prospective meta-analyses of genome-wide association studies from 5 cohorts. *Circ Cardiovasc Genet*. 2009; **2**(1): 73–80.

10

Carrying a Center of Excellence through a Critical Transition in Leadership

The Story of the Department of Veterans Affairs HSR&D Center of Excellence on Implementing Evidence-Based Practice

Michael Weiner,[*†] *Michelle P. Salyers,*[*‡] *and Linda S. Williams*[*†]

> ### *Michael Weiner's Story of a Success in Science*
>
> I recall facing a challenge in the merger of a funded research activity with a clinical improvement task force's charge to improve the quality of referrals. These two activities were happening in parallel initially, but we were able to integrate them because we realized that our goals were actually the same. In one corner of the project we were working with a team of clinicians who

* Center of Excellence on Implementing Evidence-Based Practice, Department of Veterans Affairs, Veterans Health Administration, Health Services Research and Development Service HFP 04-148.
Center for Health Services Research, Regenstrief Institute, Inc.
Indiana University Center for Health Services and Outcomes Research.
† Indiana University School of Medicine.
‡ School of Science, Indiana University-Purdue University Indianapolis, Indianapolis, Indiana, United States.

faced a problem with information and requests that were getting lost in the referral-consultation process. This was in the outpatient setting and so we needed a way to develop an approach to fix that problem. It was going to be difficult because there were people from specialty care and primary care involved, and these individuals didn't know each other very well. It was a diverse group – an endocrinologist, primary care physician, an informatician, representatives of hospital administration, and me (the health services researcher and research-minded team member). The work was challenging for a few reasons. One was just the different kind of work flows we were trying to coordinate and integrate. Another was probably some preconceived differences of opinions about roles, especially differing opinions about who should play what role in the clinical process. For example, if I refer a patient to a specialist, who is actually responsible for setting up an appointment, the specialist or the referring primary care generalist? Does this responsibility lie with the referring team that follows the patient or with the specialist? Should the specialist call the patient and arrange a calendar? Low-level decisions like this become important in trying to support a process. The fact that we had very different expectations and opinions about how it should work meant that we had to have many discussions just to identify optimal work flow. We were also trying to implement a new informatics product and to develop this product we had to have a working plan for its implementation. The implementation process had to be co-developed in an interactive process engaging this whole team of stakeholders. It was challenging for a researcher who was not a lead clinician. As a researcher I was in a situation where I was trying to bring my knowledge and information from evidence to bear on this clinical scenario but wasn't really in charge of the clinical environment. By working within this team and sharing goals we converged on a definition of the problem and how we wanted to address it. We were able to stimulate some useful changes and introduce a new tool to alleviate the problem.

Introduction

In this chapter, we discuss a transition in leadership that occurred in a research center of excellence funded by the US Department of Veterans Affairs, housed in a large medical center located on an urban university campus. All research centers undergo periodic transitions in leadership – some of which are more successful than others. In some circumstances but not all, these transitions are planned and managed. Transition is often necessitated when an institution establishes new priorities and directions that affect the center favorably or unfavorably. In our case, concurrent changes in funding and key personnel made the transition more challenging and complex.

Our story begins with the unexpected transition of a leader at a time when an application for renewal of core research funding was imminent. We describe how the transition evolved, key decisions were made, new leaders were identified, and the factors that were considered most important in moving the Center forward. We describe who we are, what we do, and what was happening in our Center at the time of the transition. We then discuss initial events, interim leadership, and how the Center pursued a major renewal of funding during the same period. The process of recruiting a new Director during this period of uncertainty is discussed. Building internal and external relationships is addressed, followed by management of the "hand-off" to the new leader. These sections detail how the research center was preserved and ultimately strengthened. We end with discussion, reflection, and lessons learned from our experiences.

We believe our "case study in change" will be most useful to students of the organizational culture of research centers, and the administrators, institutional leaders, and collaborators who interact with them. It may be particularly relevant for those who are engaged in, or foresee, a transition in their own environment. We hope that through this work, qualities and characteristics of successful leadership transitions, as well as some of the costs of challenging transitions, will become better understood.

Background/Scenario

Our research center, the VA Health Services Research and Development (HSR&D) Center of Excellence on Implementing Evidence-Based Practice (CIEBP), is based at the Richard L. Roudebush VA Medical Center in Indianapolis, Indiana. Like all other VA HSR&D Centers, we underwent annual reviews, with the opportunity to compare our individual Center with aggregate data from other Centers. Metrics of success for the annual review included assessments of: the number of grants, funding source, and total grant award amounts held by Center investigators, the number of publications and presentations by Center investigators, and specific impacts of our research on Veterans or the VA health-care system. This last metric reflects the innovative nature of the VA health-care system and makes our Center somewhat different from many other academic research centers; that is, a VA HSR&D Center is expected to generate new research products as well as strategic improvements in VA health care.

At the time of this leadership transition in 2008, our Center was four years old and was focused on improving health care by studying methods of adopting, disseminating, and sustaining best practices among a range of disciplines. During the first few years of our Center's life, much of our activity centered on recruiting exceptional MD and PhD health services researchers and on increasing the number of VA and non-VA funded research projects held by our core investigators. We had experienced considerable success in recruiting, adding 14 new investigators in the first three years with concomitant increases in the number of research projects and staff.

Although rapid growth was clearly fundamental to our success, it resulted in a diversity of research interests that did not always have a clear, coherent focus. In contrast to other research centers with a disease-based focus, our focus on implementation of evidence led to the recruitment of a wide range of investigators from many different scientific backgrounds. For example, during the first few years, we added several junior MD health services researchers with diverse clinical research interests (cancer, mental health, pain), and PhD investigators from fields like psychology, organizational development, communication, and human factors engineering. We also made progress during this time in increasing the total number of VA-funded research projects, but given the fact that this metric necessarily lags recruitment of junior investigators by about two years, at the time of our leadership change, we were among the VA HSR&D Centers with the lowest number of VA HSR&D funded grants.

All VA HSR&D Centers are required to re-compete for another five-year term of funding at the beginning of the fourth year. The timing of our renewal application coincided directly with the leadership change. This change in circumstance created several unique vulnerabilities for our Center. First, it generated immediate questions among investigators about the prospects for renewed funding as a Center. Junior investigators who were planning to apply for, or had recently received, career development awards were especially vulnerable, because they depended on the Center's core resources to support their career development and pilot projects. The announcement also generated concerns among staff about job stability and continuity of relationship with other Center members. Among research teams, the leadership change in some ways created a "bunker mentality," where team members were tempted to focus exclusively on what they could do to ensure their own survival rather than spend their collective effort on a potentially unsuccessful Center renewal application. Because VA HSR&D Centers exist in relationship to one or more VA medical centers, there were also concerns among Center investigators that we would be unable to secure the space and resource commitments from our facility's administration, to demonstrate strong local support for our renewal application and to provide the necessary resources to continue growing. At this same time, the Center also developed vacancies for the Administrative Officer and Senior Program Manager positions, creating concerns about overall staffing levels. With less than 3 months from the time of the leadership change to the application date, we had to address the changes and their potential implications quickly and directly.

Key Areas of Activity/Focus

Leadership Transition

At the time of leadership change, there was no clear successor in the Center. There were relatively few senior researchers with administrative experience, and those with appointments to the Center were all fully funded. At the same time, several junior researchers who lacked full funding and thus would have time to do research administration (0.5 FTE devoted to Center administration per VA regulation) were too early in their careers to assume major administrative responsibilities. An executive council, which had been formed several months earlier and included the Center's new Associate Director, other center investigators, and local research and administrative partners, held a series of meetings to identify a plan for leadership transition and to address the issue of who could effectively lead the center as we searched for a permanent Director. After several meetings, two of us (LW and MS) discussed the possibility of sharing the role of interim Director. This made sense from several perspectives. First, at different times in its history each of us had been Associate Directors of the Center and we were familiar with its processes and procedures. Both of us had a stable track record of funding, had leadership responsibilities within our own research programs, and had excellent research teams in place. Recognizing the challenges taking on additional responsibilities would entail, each of us went through a process of careful reflection and consideration. For example, LW conducted a concept mapping exercise to identify positive, negative, and neutral impacts on core "assets," including her research program/team, individual research career, clinical role as a staff physician, and family. To make time to fill the 0.50 FTE combined position, each of us had to give up other responsibilities. LW reduced her clinical administrative responsibilities, stepping down as Chief of Neurology, and MS was able to increase her availability in the Center by cutting back on responsibilities at the university. Finally, and perhaps most importantly, our discussions reinforced a deep sense of trust and commitment to one another and to the task at hand.

As acting co-Directors, we divided responsibilities among ourselves and the Center's Associate Director. LW led the Center in external relations and finance; MS led internal organizational development and post-award resource management (e.g., personnel, space, and work flow). The Associate Director oversaw fellowships, hiring, information technology, and issues pertaining to data management and security. We met weekly to coordinate efforts, and developed an e-mail-based communication system for rapid identification of issues that needed action. Having separate but coordinated leadership roles allowed us to manage center operations efficiently while maintaining our ongoing research commitments.

The shared leadership model was broadened to facilitate key activities in other Center operations. For example, we created volunteer workgroups in finance, post-award resources, fellowships, organizational development, and faculty recruitment to improve participation and effectiveness of the Center's activities. Groups met weekly or biweekly, to evaluate current operations, plan for ongoing activities, and resolve concerns. Each workgroup communicated their activities to a specific member of the team, who then brought items of interest or discussion to the Center's interim leaders. Creating shared leadership[1] in multi-stakeholder workgroups paralleled our own process and confirmed some of our own organizational change research findings.

Funding Renewal

Our first major leadership challenge was crafting a successful renewal proposal for our Center in a very short period of time. In fact, these discussions predated the actual leadership change as senior investigators and Center advisors worked to develop a strategy for maximizing our success in securing renewed funding. Early discussions focused on optimal timing for the leadership transition. Although some believed that the chances were best if the change occurred after the renewal proposal was submitted, we concluded that making the change prior to submitting the proposal was more accurate and transparent. It also had the advantage of establishing the roles of the interim leaders and engaging the Center's investigators in the shared task of securing renewal funding.

The decision to change leadership before submitting the renewal application set the tone for the content and process of writing. We sought feedback from multiple stakeholders on the story of the leadership transition; this was a key section of the application that we knew would be fundamental to our review. In this section, the many accomplishments of the previous leader and the positive reasons underlying the leadership change at a somewhat unusual point were highlighted. Explicit plans for interim leadership and management of the Center during the process of recruiting a permanent Director were detailed. A key aspect of this story was the strong ongoing relationship of the Center with our Medical Center administration and academic partners. This positive relationship was described in the application and in accompanying supporting letters, and was made evident by new commitments (financial, space, and personnel) to the Center. Because the interim co-Director structure was atypical, we also expressly described our management plan for key Center functions and how our co-Director roles worked within the organizational management structure of the Center and our parent medical facility. It was important that this section be transparent and thoughtful in reassuring reviewers about the co-Directors' and our partners' unwavering commitment to the mission, goals and products of the Center, regardless of the time and other resources needed to recruit a new Director.

The process of writing a five-year proposal with a $1 million annual core budget was daunting. Without this core funding for infrastructure, support for the grants manager, Associate Director, program support assistants, Administrative Officer (the lead administrator), other key staff, equipment, and the Steering Committee would disappear. In retrospect, writing the proposal served as a key activity that promoted immediate engagement of many stakeholders in determining our strategic focus and direction. From the beginning the renewal was framed as a "sprint" activity, as distinct from other management and leadership activities that were more "marathon" in nature. A draft of strategic foci and aims for the Center was shared with investigators in a series of town-hall meetings to seek feedback and modification of our drafts. Once investigators agreed upon core themes, they self-identified with independent workgroups around core themes to further refine the aims and plan projects within each area of focus. Each workgroup was charged with identifying three-year and five-year strategic goals with details about how they would be achieved and what metrics would be used to measure success in each area. These activities brought people together to talk about how they saw themselves and their work fitting best into the Center, promoted better understanding of individual lines of research, stimulated new collaborations, and created shared energy around the ability of individuals to influence what our Center could become.

The Center's co-Directors, both of whom were experienced grant writers, explicitly divided writing tasks between themselves and other key investigators and staff. One person led the writing of the strategic plan and research foci sections; the other took responsibility for the key accomplishments, personnel, and resources sections. With barely 6 weeks to complete, a timeline was developed by the co-Directors and supported by all key contributors. This included hard deadlines for section drafts, full drafts, and a detailed internal review schedule. All investigators were offered the opportunity to sign up as reviewers, and assignments were made based on investigators' availability according to the specific timeline. For example, one investigator would sign up to get the draft on a specific day and to give edits of the draft to the next reviewer by another given day. This process produced a high-quality draft relatively quickly and also empowered investigators and staff to put forward their best contributions. Finally, input from outside reviewers familiar with our work and the funding agency was also sought and was instrumental in successfully crafting our message.

Once the hurdle of the initial review was cleared, preparations took place for a site visit that the funding agency requested. The Center's leaders prepared investigators and partners for this interaction, organizing a plan for the site visit to demonstrate a clear, strong line of support and commitment from all involved. Meetings were held to discuss the structure of the site visit and the messages to be emphasized. To facilitate open conversations, the site visit was arranged with a series of conversations between the site reviewers and key groups, including the Center's leaders, investigators, staff, and partners, giving ample opportunity for the reviewers to seek specific information from various stakeholders. This approach highlighted our existing areas of expertise, the engagement of our investigators and staff in our core mission, the relational strength between the Center's leaders and partners, and ultimately our ability to thrive during an abrupt leadership transition and beyond.

Ultimately, our efforts were rewarded with a one-year renewal of funding – with the remaining years of funding contingent upon successful recruitment of a permanent Director. Thus, only part of our work was complete.

Recruiting in an Uncertain Time

At the same time that leadership changed and the search for a new Director began, the Center was faced with additional recruiting needs. Several key administrative staff had recently left and the Center had a large number of active investigators requiring ongoing administrative support and mentorship. What sort of individual would consider taking on a key administrative role or directorship of a center with uncertainty about funding and many other pressing needs? This would most likely be an individual who would view the position as a high-risk, high-gain opportunity for career advancement and a chance to help the Center grow and become stronger. As a somewhat risky proposition, it would not be likely to be a good fit for someone with a high need for control or established stability and order.

A potentially useful analogy is to think of the Center as the seller, and the Director-candidate as the buyer. In this scenario, a key assessment for the buyer includes the current and future value of the proposition. In our case, the Center was undervalued because it had talented investigators and staff, with excellent track records in research – but was currently in a position risking their momentum via loss of supportive funding. An undervalued Center could provide satisfaction and professional reward to the candidate willing to invest in change. Recruitment in this situation had to focus on current strengths, collaborations, and accomplishments, and also on potential and opportunities for growth in areas of strength. Discussions with candidates had to be frank and open but focused on bright possibilities. Acknowledging the challenges that the Center had faced, and outlining the approach and solutions that had been developed, provided a level of integrity while also generating recognition for how the leaders had pursued a difficult situation. Fortunately, all of the core investigators remained at the Center and were eager to help recruit a strong candidate. Involving investigators and staff in the candidate interview and selection process was a living embodiment of the interim leadership team's commitment to transparency and shared decision making, and further allowed investigators to solidify their own enthusiasm and commitment to their own work, the Center, and each other. This, in turn, helped to demonstrate the true value and potential of the Center to visiting candidates.

The actual recruitment process used several comprehensive strategies. First, we developed a capable search committee that included members in positions of leadership in the Center as well as facility leaders and key partners on campus. Second, we distributed formal announcements of the position opening, broadly soliciting applications widely. Third, the search committee worked with the Center's investigators and academic partners to identify local, qualified candidates with experience in similar areas who might be interested. Local candidates might be especially valuable due to their familiarity with the environment, but an external candidate could bring fresh ideas and complementary skills. Personal invitations were extended to candidates of interest encouraging them to consider applying.

One critical element that aided in recruitment was securing commitments of financial support and additional space from the facility's leaders prior to launching the search. Regardless of the outcome of the Center's renewal application, the Medical Center was committed to its continued support. One potentially difficult situation arose when the Medical Center instituted a hiring freeze during the time of recruitment. Because of the multiple open positions in the Center, this situation could have been disastrous. Working with the Medical Center's leaders, however, we confirmed that a hiring freeze would not affect us if we clearly identified and communicated our own line of funding (e.g., specific grants and time periods) to hire each requested position. Clarifying these issues with institutional leaders was clearly important for our recruitment efforts.

Another important aspect of the Center during recruitment was the environment. During visits, the candidate would consider the overall "tone" or atmosphere of the Center. Is it quiet or busy? Do people look anxious or confident? Did we create a public forum for intellectual discourse that provided a "safe" environment and also promoted the highest degree of scientific rigor? Candidates commented favorably on this, inspiring confidence that investing in the Center was worthwhile.

After identifying several potential candidates for Director, we held a series of in-person interviews. In trying to attract a candidate under challenging circumstances it might have been tempting to focus only on the positive aspects of the organization. Although we tried to accommodate the candidates' interests, we also made clear the collectively derived expectations and responsibilities that were necessary to meet the Center's needs. Given the recently funded renewal application, it was important that the future Director be able to align his or her plans with the stated strategic plan, at least in the near term. A candidate's desire to take the Center in a radically new direction would have been in conflict with our leadership approach at the time and would have made it difficult for us to meet our stated goals and metrics.

The recruitment of other key staff generally followed a similar direction, though tailored to the needs of those positions. One particular difficulty was the VA requirement for US citizenship, which made hiring statisticians especially difficult, since many graduates with statistics degrees are not US citizens. Addressing this required creativity, to identify ways to streamline the system or find acceptable alternatives, such as short-term contracting with our university or use of alternative funding streams. Discussion of this issue with Director-applicants helped to provide reassurance that the issue was being reviewed and addressed thoughtfully.

Internal Community Building/Relationships

During the leadership transition, we wanted to ensure an ongoing sense of community within the Center. Because a change of leadership and a renewal application can bring uncertainty and even fear, we focused a great deal of effort on providing a sense of stability and consistency, with clear communication and access. We felt that an explicit focus on strengthening ties among the Center's staff and investigators could go far in creating a calming, connected workplace. To promote this atmosphere, we made decisions transparent, posting minutes from leadership meetings, as well as minutes from all workgroups so that everyone in the Center could read directly what was happening. We held Center-wide meetings to discuss transition plans and answer questions. We held office hours each week so that staff and investigators had a consistent time to ask questions or seek assistance directly from leaders. We also coordinated travel plans so that a leadership team member was always on site. As noted earlier, self-organizing workgroups were developed to focus on core Center activities, and these groups may have helped the Center's members feel connected to others through regular meetings and a shared mission.

A particularly important and exciting work group was the organizational development team, led by one staff member and one investigator, both of whom were longtime Center members. The group met biweekly to discuss and resolve issues related to morale. This workgroup planned a series of short retreats – a half-day and several 2-hour meetings – that included team-building exercises, along with didactic topics that were deemed important by the group (e.g., managing conflict, addressing gossip, dealing with change). The organizational development group also sponsored a pitch-in (pot luck) picnic lunch and reinstated monthly birthday celebrations.

The organizational development workgroup also created a mechanism for engaging and welcoming new staff into the center. They created a welcome packet that included photos and information about existing staff and investigators, and a buddy system to pair an existing staff member with the new person so that they would have a go-to person should they need assistance. The buddy was also responsible for introducing the new staff member to others in the Center, and periodically checking in to help ensure successful integration and help problem solve where necessary.

External Community Building/Relationships

Another key aspect of both the renewal application and our leadership transition was cultivating relationships with key external partners. We already had an established steering committee of national health services research experts, who visited annually to engage in discussions about strengths, weaknesses, and strategies for growth and improvement. We quickly turned to this group after the initial leadership change occurred, to help us consider various options for describing the Center and our approach to the renewal. This was extremely helpful, since we obtained "high-level advice" from experienced people who knew us and knew the review process for renewal. In addition, we met face to face with several committee members and also held a series of conference calls to review our developing renewal proposal.

Our two closest and most important external partners were our parent VA Medical Center and our long-standing local partner, Regenstrief Institute, Inc., which is a center of our academic affiliate, the Indiana University School of Medicine. We worked very closely with leaders from these organizations throughout the leadership transition, the renewal process, and the ongoing process of the Center's management and recruitment. Leaders from these organizations joined our weekly Executive Council meetings, allowing frequent communication and discussion on short- and long-term issues. We knew that strong relationships with these partners were key to our success, and we worked to establish reciprocal trust and shared goals. We implemented an agreement with our Medical Center to have use of a portion of the indirect funds generated by our research. We also detailed a process by which we would submit an annual budget request for accessing these funds and jointly review budget needs throughout the year so that unused funds could be targeted to support other needs in the facility. This forthright negotiation ensured that all parties agreed that the ultimate success of the Center was a component of the overall success and health of our Medical Center.

We also successfully negotiated with our Medical Center to have an experienced financial administrator assigned to our Center for several months as we recruited a lead administrator. This helped us accomplish critical administrative work in the Center, and brought new shared understanding between us as researchers and our Medical Center partners. This "cultural exchange" resulted in much more effective communication as we learned to speak and hear each other's language, know the pressures and expectations that we each faced, and learned that there were many ways in which we could help each other to be successful.

Managing the Hand-off Transition to a New Director

Our recruitment strategy paid off and the search for a new Director proved successful. The incoming Director worked for the academic affiliate, knew the campus and environment, but was not currently employed by the VA. His major research interest was health informatics, a core area for growth in the Center. In keeping with the principle of community practice, the interim leadership team held regular meetings with the incoming Director before his official appointment began. This allowed the team to discuss active issues and encouraged input from interim and incoming leaders to shape decisions being made during this period. After the new Director officially assumed the role, he continued periodic meetings with the former leadership team, to help learn about historical perspectives and precedents. The former leadership team essentially served in an advisory role that added stability to the transition. The Associate Director, who had not shifted roles throughout this period, helped to maintain continuity and momentum of certain activities in process, such as acquisition and implementation of computer software in the Center. In addition, the Associate Director continued to reassure staff and help them to adjust to the changes at hand.

In addition to regular leadership meetings, which occurred for several months, the new Director started to meet regularly with the Center's newly hired Administrative Officer. This team progressively developed their own working approach to directing personnel and activities of the Center. Discussions included aspects of hiring, staff and investigator management, space, policies, funding and other budgetary issues, and relationships with various organizational units in the facility. A monthly Center-wide meeting with investigators and staff included updates about these topics and invited questions and open discussion.

The Director's other daily decisions also required similar attention to, and balance of, historical actions and new needs. Monthly meetings with investigators or staff were often used to review and modify policies dealing with such issues as scientific conduct, protecting data and human subjects, pursuit of new funding, work hours, and use of shared resources. Leaders and other personnel shared the desire for a fresh start, while needing to carry forward and resolve any issues around recent or ongoing collaborations. At this point, the Center had 18 investigators, five fellows, and 29 staff, with grant awards of about $4.4 million. Although the incoming Director had previously known several investigators in the Center, many were new, and there were also many staff to meet. The Director set up individual meetings with all investigators, trainees, and staff, to become better acquainted and to identify any issues that needed immediate attention.

Not everything went smoothly during these initial months. The first 6 months under the incoming Director's leadership found some lingering anxiety, primarily from staff, about the change. Communication with staff was not always as clear and as timely as it could have been. Competing needs were not always met in a timely way. This may in part be a decision-making style, but was also grounded in a deliberate desire to learn about the Center and all sides of issues before taking action. Some adjustment period was needed to instill confidence and foster clear communication in a new leadership environment.

In many organizations experiencing leadership transition, a certain amount of "shakeup" often occurs. This may involve hiring or firing of certain staff, due to misalignments of priorities or perspectives that become evident as new leaders come on board. We sought to minimize early shifts of personnel that might be considered disruptive. Nevertheless, some staff were let go during both the interim and the new leadership period for failing to adhere to core policies or achieve expected performance. This unpleasant activity is made more difficult during times of leadership transition, where assumptions about such actions may lead to harmful gossip that impacts morale. We tried to limit this by communicating clearly but with appropriate discretion that key policies must be enforced and employees are accountable for their work.

Another area of change was in our fellowship training program as training programs may be especially vulnerable during transitions. In our case, the fellowship director had multiple, competing, and new priorities. The new Center Director met several times with the Fellowship Director and the fellows, to review mentoring, curricula, resources, and fellows' progress in the program. After a period of time, we identified a new pair of co-Directors to lead and strengthen the fellowship programs.

With the hiring of many new staff, policy development and documentation was another area of growth in the early period after the transition. In many workplaces, leaders may make commitments or promises to employees, perhaps concerning salaries, bonuses, benefits, office space, or other resources. The handling of such commitments across a transition in leadership requires special attention to ensure fairness, honesty, and clear expectations. The Director conveyed and followed an intention to honor previously documented commitments to the greatest extent possible. At the same time, the leaders were motivated to improve and expand upon the Center's collection of written policies.

Finally, a Director brought from outside the institution, as in our case, lacks certain information about how the organization works. The new Director invested heavily in gaining a rapid understanding of the organization, how it worked, and what would help or hinder it. The Director openly sought such information from personnel in and around the Center. To maximize the accuracy of information gathered, multiple sources of information, rather than just one or two "preferred" sources, were found to work best. Although openly seeking information could create a certain amount of vulnerability via acknowledging an initial lack of knowledge, asking informed questions, gaining knowledge quickly, and responding to emerging issues would minimize perceptions of vulnerability, and would maximize trust and engagement among personnel.

Discussion

We are fortunate that our Center was successful during this leadership transition. We were able to maintain our full status as a research center of excellence, with five years of new funding awarded. We were able to recruit a new Director in a relatively short period of time (14 months). Notably, none of the investigators, including those recruited by the previous Director, left during this time, and we recruited additional investigators, fellows, and staff to continue growth. With the benefit of hindsight, time, and shared perspectives, we recognize several key themes that we believe were critical to our success.

One overarching theme is the *commitment of leaders who believed in the Center's value and future.* This was true of the interim and permanent directors, and also leadership of our partner organizations and members of our Center. Interim leaders were willing to devote a substantial amount of time and energy, and did so because we were committed to the Center's success and believed that the Center would continue to prosper. After we began the interim role, we became aware of the "glass cliff" phenomenon. This term refers to the observation that once the glass ceiling of attaining a leadership position has been broken, women are more likely than men to be chosen as leaders in high-risk or failing organizations.[2] Empiric research about this phenomenon has identified some possible explanations, including the observation that characteristics more often associated with women than men in the workplace (e.g., improved people management, empathy, and communication skills) may be valued more highly in times of crisis than leadership characteristics more typically associated with men (e.g. decisiveness). Furthermore, this tendency to ascribe gender stereotypes to leadership candidates may be increased specifically during times of perceived crisis.[3,4] In our case, although identified by others as potential candidates for Center leadership, we (MS and LW, both women) crafted and proposed this shared leadership role. There may have been some temporary changes in some aspects of our professional work (e.g., fewer first author publications during the time of the transition and shared leadership); however, we believe this role did not negatively affect our careers. To the contrary, we have learned a great deal and have been able to translate that learning into our improvements in our ongoing research leadership roles. When interim leaders are needed, however, consideration of how and why specific leaders are being suggested should be encouraged.

Our Center's relationship with leaders in our partner organizations was critical. They expressed their commitment by actively participating in regular meetings with our Center, providing instrumental support in terms of funding, space, and personnel, and advocating on our behalf during the Center's renewal site visit. These visible and clear commitments helped to provide additional reassurance to engage a Director candidate, and they ultimately led to strengthened collaboration and understanding between the Center and its partners. In addition, a core panel of leaders in the form of the executive council provided a sense of stability for the Center.

We believe that *shared leadership throughout the Center* was important to our success. Hecker and Birla assert that "empowerment and the ability to create leaders at every level are central to effective leadership."[5] Distributing leadership responsibility should involve mobilizing personnel to generate solutions.[1] Input from internal stakeholders can help to reduce burnout and improve morale. Self-determination theory is built on the premise that human potential is at its best when we have autonomy, mastery, and connectedness.[6] By creating self-organizing workgroups, people could connect with each other and contribute to leading the Center in areas of their interest and expertise. At the outset, we also clearly understood that to take on an additional leadership role meant making choices about what activities we would have to modify (at least for the time being). We also had to consider who would be impacted by these choices, and what we could do to minimize any disruption in ongoing activities and relationships. In our experience, this honest self-appraisal is not always undertaken by individuals contemplating leadership roles, and it is not always encouraged by organizations who may naturally seek to get "more for less." However, this sort of thoughtful appraisal is fundamental to the success of any new major activity that one contemplates taking on as part of their research career.

Further, quality improvement research has shown that involving all types of staff when designing improvements results in greater success of the improvement activity.[7,8] We should note, however, that not all members of the Center believed that this was the right approach. Some staff expressed concerns that a shared leadership style that invited input from all levels was potentially destructive and instead advocated for a more top-down, hierarchical approach with clearer lines of communication. In times of crisis, an authoritarian leadership style may be preferred. Perhaps it is a sense of structure that is important during crisis. We tried to instill this through regular meetings, consistent presence, and a clear division of responsibilities, while also encouraging autonomy. Although we are part of the VA, we also reside and work in an academic setting, where autonomy is highly valued. Conflicting cultures within a single organization may require unusual balance and leadership strategies, but can be addressed with discussion about potential management strategies and with transparency about management decisions.

Throughout our transition, we paid special attention to maintaining a high level of *clear communication*. We believed that this helped to reduce anxiety, by providing a sense of predictability and perceived control during stressful times. Posting minutes of leadership meetings and workgroups, having frequent all-staff meetings, and regular opportunities to speak directly with leadership were important methods for us. Our ability to do this successfully relied on our intentional efforts to ensure clear communication among the interim leaders so we could avoid giving mixed messages to Center investigators and staff, and finally among the interim leaders and the incoming Director.

What is perhaps the most unifying theme of all is that *a successful center is built from strong relationships*. Reflecting successful medical practice, a relationship-centered approach became the foundation of our Center. This concept of relationship-centered leadership traits has also been identified as a core component of an emerging non-traditional model of leadership.[9] Relational transparency has been described as a key component of authentic leadership.[10] Although the interim leadership team all knew one another, we had to invest in developing strong relationships as co-leaders in order to meet the challenge of the leadership transition. Our staff had to work to bridge potential gulfs between existing research teams and perceived distinctions between types of staff members to support our overall success. Our organizational development team fundamentally took relationship-centered organization as its mission in creating opportunities to connect, expand, and grow in the Center. Finally, when our new Director joined the Center, one of his first efforts was meeting all Center members to establish his own relationships with them. These activities, occurring at all levels of our Center, clearly reflect the importance and value of relationship to supporting teams through a leadership transition.

Conclusion

Change is undeniably stressful. In today's climate of shrinking research funding, increased competition for funds, and often tenuous academic support for research, the ability to sustain an academic research enterprise is dependent on the ability of its leaders to successfully manage change. Based on our experience, and even in trying circumstances, change can be not just managed but used as a catalyst to promote improvement. With core commitment from leaders to *investing* in the value of the research unit rather than individual pursuits, *sharing* leadership across traditional boundaries, *communicating* clearly with other leaders and with all personnel, and to *building* strong relationships with colleagues and partners, we are confident that even in times of change improved culture and performance of academic research units can surely be achieved.

Acknowledgments

We are grateful to the VA HSR&D program and its Center of Excellence on Implementing Evidence-Based Practice. We also thank our informal reviewers, including Laurie Plue. The work reported here was supported by the Department of Veterans Affairs, Veterans Health Administration, Health Services Research and Development Service HFP 04-148. Dr. Weiner is Chief of Health Services Research and Development at the Richard L. Roudebush Veterans Affairs Medical Center in Indianapolis, Indiana, United States. The views expressed in this work are those of the authors and do not necessarily represent the views of the Department of Veterans Affairs.

References

1. Heifetz R, Grashow A, Linsky M. Leadership in a (permanent) crisis. *Harvard Business Review.* 2009; **87**(7–8): 62–9, 153. Epub 2009/07/28.
2. Ryan MK, Haslam SA. The glass cliff: evidence that women are over-represented in precarious leadership positions. *Br J Management.* 2005; **16**: 81–90.
3. Ryan MK, Haslam SA. The glass cliff: exploring the dynamics surrounding the appointment of women to precarious leadership positions. *Acad Management Rev.* 2007; **32**: 549–72.
4. Bruckmuller S, Branscombe NR. The glass cliff: when and why women are selected as leaders in crisis contexts. *Br J Soc Psychol.* 2010; **49**(Pt 3): 433–51. Epub 2009/08/21.
5. Hecker L, Birla RK. Intangible factors leading to success in research: strategy, innovation and leadership. *J Cardiovasc Transl Res.* 2008; **1**(1): 85–92. Epub 2008/03/01.

6. Ryan RM, Deci EL. Self-determination theory and the facilitation of intrinsic motivation, social development, and well-being. *Am Psychol*. 2000; **55**(1): 68–78. Epub 2001/06/08.
7. Nelson EC, Batalden PB, Huber TP, *et al*. Microsystems in health care: Part 1. Learning from high-performing front-line clinical units. *Jt Comm J Qual Improv*. 2002; **28**(9): 472–93. Epub 2002/09/10.
8. Wang MC, Hyun JK, Harrison M, *et al*. Redesigning health systems for quality: lessons from emerging practices. *Jt Comm J Qual Patient Saf*. 2006; **32**(11): 599–611. Epub 2006/11/24.
9. Cheung FM, Halpern DF. Women at the top: powerful leaders define success as work + family in a culture of gender. *Am Psychol*. 2010; **65**(3): 182–93. Epub 2010/03/31.
10. Avolio BJ, Walumbwa FO, Weber TJ. Leadership: current theories, research, and future directions. *Annu Rev Psychol*. 2009; **60**: 421–49. Epub 2008/07/25.

11

Epilogue and Look Forward

Richard M. Frankel and Thomas S. Inui

***Thomas Inui Discovers the Process of Research Inquiry: Sephadex,
My Sephadex***

Forty years ago, medical schools favored the admission of persons with liberal arts backgrounds. At the same time they also implemented programs to assure a significant exposure for each medical student to one or another of the basic sciences of our discipline during the preclinical curriculum.

I entered medical school fresh from a background as an undergraduate philosophy major, flush with enthusiasm for the power of careful thought and rigorous analysis (research), ready for wrestling with the real problems of sick people. Pre-Socratics, Plato, Kant, Kierkegaard and 20th-century existentialist literature – this odyssey had been my intellectual coming-of-age, signaled by a note home in midcourse, "Dear Mom and Dad: Just a line to let you know I've decided to major in philosophy. Don't worry. I've got a practical minor – religion!" It had been an exhilarating experience, no doubt the optimal preparation for medical school. The choice of majors was my own, fortunately, not just what the admissions doctor ordered, since the lack of a substantial undergraduate background in basic science certainly extracted a great price over the next two years.

Baltimore was still steamy hot that late summer when we all arrived, eyeing one another with trepidation and suspicion. The Hopkins curriculum was fashioned into "blocks," 10-week segments entirely devoted to intensive experiences in physiologic chemistry, histology, neuroanatomy, and so on. Time was set aside within each block for research. At the very beginning, in physiologic chemistry, I was assigned to a partner for "independent research" in the laboratory. At last, the real stuff, a white (knee-length) lab coat, and an experienced partner (biochemistry major) for buoyancy. Our faculty mentor presented us with a murky flask of *Escherichia coli*, instructions for growing them, methods for preparing and "harvesting" (wonderful language, bringing home the sheaves) membrane fractionates, as well as a description of an assay procedure for a membranebound ATPase. The latter enzyme, by his prior work, was probably a sodium pump, calcium-stimulated, magnesium-inhibited, but inadequately characterized. Our task was to produce a much-purified form of the enzyme for further work. The approach was simple, he said. We simply needed to find the right Sephadex.

I knew nothing of Sephadex, but we became intimately acquainted. It was gritty stuff, as I recall, said to have "pores" of differing size. You grew the bacteria, went to the cold room, centrifuged, suspended, Waring-blenderized at length, recentrifuged, resuspended, and dripped the suspension slowly through a column of Sephadex into a fractionating collector. Finally, out of the cold, the tubes were assayed, one by one, for the presence of the ATPase. The deeper the purple hue, the more enzyme present. By luck of the draw, my role was played out largely in the cold room. Jacketed, I spent every spare waking hour there, emerging from time to time to squint through steamed-up glasses at colorimetric assay data. In the end we succeeded, the tubes turned nearly as purple as my fingers and lips. My partner forged his now white-hot interest in basic research into a career in physiologic chemistry. I left "the bench" with no regrets, seeking more temperate intellectual climes.

It was later that I rediscovered the special rewards of inquiry and discovery. In my instance, the problems and questions of greatest interest occurred naturally and in great profusion, like thickets of thistles, in the context of clinical care, particularly on an ambulatory basis. I developed a special affinity for studying health-related behaviors, since so many of the problems seemed behavioral at their crux. Warming to the tasks of research required rediscovery of research as a problem-solving enterprise, not the mindless application and reapplication of known methods, whatever their merits, elegance, or power.

Inui TS. Sephadex, my Sephadex: discovering the process of inquiry. *Soc Gen Intern Med Newsletter*. 1987; **10**(5): 2. Reprinted with permission *SGIM*.

The word research first came into use in France in 1588. It literally means to re-search, (old French re-, *re-* + cerchier, *to search*).[1] In 17th-century England the term was part of a phrase "to search and research," meaning to look carefully. In modern times, the word has perhaps lost a bit of the sense of re-doubling one's efforts, although "Sephadex, my Sephadex" illustrates the fact that much of basic laboratory science derives from careful searching and re-searching for answers to puzzling questions. As researchers, ourselves, in a particular place, time and academic health science center, the "puzzle" with which we began as we contemplated this volume was wanting to learn from a diverse set of authors from different countries, and in different health science centers around the world, what their experiences in conducting and promoting research in academic health sciences centers had been. And, given our backgrounds and interests as "social" scientists, we were also curious to know about the "stories behind the stories;" that is, the personal stories of these scientists and what it was that motivated them to do what they did and didn't do. In both pursuits, our re-searching was richly rewarded.

What did we learn? First, we learned that in most cases, there was little that separated the personal from the professional in the stories we heard. Deep personal commitments to success and scientific advance lived side by side. In some cases it was a belief in self-actualization, in other cases a belief in helping others succeed, and in still other cases it was a belief in the future of a country or its citizenry. Understanding the connection between the personal and the professional is helpful in bringing to life the larger picture within which scientific research occurs. By convention, most scientific writing is devoid of personal biography and the motivation, energy, and desire that lead to searching and re-searching problems large and small. As described above, one might have the desire and drive to be a re-searcher and discover that the problems of bench chemistry may resonate with one person but not another. We learned from our "appreciative" interviews that many of the researchers who contributed to this volume followed paths that were emergent – journeys that unfolded non-linearly – and were the product of trial and error, although this would be hard to discern from simply reading their personal biography of scientific publications.

Second, we learned that despite intense pressure to compete, communitarian values are a main ingredient in the success of the scientists and the academic health science centers in which many of them work. For example, we learned of efforts in China to democratize the use of laboratory equipment so that multiple researchers might gain access to equipment they could otherwise not afford on their own. This approach also ensured optimal use of equipment that might lie fallow for long periods of time. From the same author we learned about efforts to raise research standards for an entire country by thinking collectively about manpower needs and how to achieve them. And, although the context was vastly different in some ways, we learned from the director of federally funded clinical and translational science award (CTSA) how the initial rejection of the academic health science center's proposal led to the emergence of community in the successful re-submission process.

Third, we learned that qualities of the heart such as compassion, commitment to sharing and investing in one another's success are as important as qualities of the mind that lead to success in research. We learned that the leaders of a highly successful research group were, from the beginning, fully committed to the success of colleagues, and especially so for junior investigators. Whether through sharing the task, sometimes from the burden of proposal writing, mentoring, or creating and sharing opportunities, altruism and personal sacrifice for others was present and accounted for.

It is often said that friendship and leadership do not mix; peers and employees should remain at arm's length. Despite this admonition, we heard a number of stories in which commitment to others extended well beyond the bounds of mere collegiality and blossomed into life-long friendships. In our own relationship-centered care research network, for example, we took the unusual step of engaging an expert in community formation to help create a common bond and purpose among a group of highly successful individual researchers. The result was a stunning lack of individual ego and competition among the group members and the development of close personal ties as well as high-quality research.

What does the future hold? We are encouraged by the generosity of spirit that fills these pages: generosity within and across generations of scientists and transitions in leadership; generosity that extends beyond the "business of research" into the lives and relationships of researchers to one another. We believe that much of what we have documented is being reproduced in other health science centers around the world and may well be a formula for future success. Even where it does not seem to be occurring within an academic health science center we have seen how a dedicated researcher can use his energy and influence externally to train young investigators to be mindful of the importance of community and relationships as they take up positions in academic health science centers in Japan.

As we look forward to the future, there are aspects of productive research that are likely to endure, such as the following.

● Immersion and close observation: at root, all researchers are "naturalists" and benefit from their ability to "appreciate through close observation" of the phenomena with which they work. Free association and intuitive thinking after immersion in the phenomena, perhaps even in a liminal state of mind, often is the source of inspiration and creative thought.

- Teamwork: as the personal stories in this volume attest, personal and professional relationships within teams are the source of creative energy, resiliency, expanded capacity, and fresh discovery.
- Positive challenge and disputation: challenging one another's ideas, inferences, and conclusions has long been the scientific "skeptic's" best method for arriving at "truth." In science, all conclusions are apt to be temporary and subject to future challenges, paradigm shifts, and reinterpretation. A short cut to this process of revision over time occurs within a team, through disputation and positive challenge.
- Transdisciplinary work: in science as in other endeavors, creativity may be most apt to take place in the "space between" deep disciplines or traditions of knowledge. This kind of bridge-building requires effort, trust, and mutual respect, but may be the activity in which new ideation is maximized.
- Emphasis on translation: science in the public interest requires translation from ideas and theories to applications and general use in society. While no one would dispute the value of basic science, finding ways to advance laboratory or other forms of basic research to applications with social value is one of the obligations of scientists whose work is largely supported by public funding.
- Emphasis on promoting the ideas and careers of the rising generation of scientists: mentorship and the creation of opportunities for young scientists is one of the cherished traditions and privileges of research in all domains. Working with younger scientists is invigorating and likely to sustain the careers of senior mentors. Many of the best ideas in a research career may arise and be pursued early in the career before risk-averseness and incrementalism begins to dull the edge of scientific acumen.

Other aspects of productive research, on the other hand, are likely to be subject to substantial change in the future. These might include the following.

- More interdisciplinary teamwork that links scientists with generalists: in many applied industries, generalists lead teams of subspecialists in the work of translation to products. Subspecialists and subspecialty expertise are essential, for example, in the manufacture of aerotechnology and aircraft. The management of teamwork and facilitation of role assignment and task-sharing in such teams, however, is often the function of a generalist who "keeps his/her eye on the desirable qualities of the final product" when integrating the skills, expertise, and decision making of specialists.

- Media of communication: the evolution of the Internet, means of sharing information in real time and asynchronously, and even virtual experimentation are apt to change as new modalities of data-sharing and communication infrastructure emerge. Today's applications for teleconferencing, task-sharing, and multi-tasking in dispersed environments will seem rudimentary in another 10 years. What might be possible beyond that time horizon can only be a matter for speculation and dreams. These new modalities will permit highly geographically dispersed core teams to function together and may permit global work to occur continuously as it passes from team to team in different geographic locations.

- Our models of phenomena in nature, both biologic and non-biologic, are apt to move in the direction of complexity science. As productive as the Newtonian linear models of science have been, at least half of nature is best understood to be complex responsive processes with emergent phenomena, radical interdependencies, resonance and harmonics, and unpredictability. Models of these phenomena need to advance in order to understand such basic matters as turbulence, amplification, resilience, and adaptation in biologic and social systems of relevance to health.

- Measurement technologies: in our own lifetime, we have witnessed a revolution in observation and measurement in human biology. At the beginning of our careers, x-ray crystallography and electron microscopy were revolutionary in their contributions to understanding cells and complex molecular structures like DNA. As bioengineering advances rapidly in the direction of nanotechnology, similar breakthroughs in our ability to observe and immerse ourselves in phenomena will undoubtedly occur.

- Analytic approaches like data mining, modeling, and computer-based simulations are in their infancy today. As computing power advances the application of these techniques to understanding the natural world and in the conduct of experiments in a virtual environment, our capacity to understand state changes in complex responsive systems will similarly advance.

- Funding sources: today, the United States is still the only nation in the world with a National Institutes of Health. For the past 60 years this important organization, through both its programs of intramural and extramural research funding, has permitted the United States to lead the world in biomedical research and innovation. As other nations develop and accumulate the capacity for investments in the knowledge frontier in health, it is likely that organizations of similar kinds are apt to arise in other nations. To the extent that these organizations collaborate and compete in expanding the frontiers of science, the progress of research will be accelerated and broadened.

It is perhaps audacious at best, foolish at worst, to suggest that this volume represents a new method that invites the personal to accompany the strictly scientific aspects of life and success in academic health sciences centers. At the same time there is evidence that academic institutions (including academic health science centers), in which well-being and faculty vitality are high also produce a greater return on investment.[2] Keeping considerations of what makes for excellent science and excellent relationships – that is, what gives life to academic health sciences centers – separate, may be unsustainable in the long run. Integrated research in both domains may be a key to the future health and well-being of our academic health science centers and the important work they carry out on behalf of society.

Australian Aborigines, that portion of humankind who emerged through a process of parallel evolution on a relatively isolated continent in the southern hemisphere, are said to be different from the rest of humankind in several ways. They are somewhat poikilothermic with core body temperatures that fall by several degrees during their night-time rest and sleep. They do not shiver. It is speculated that evolution in circumstances of food scarcity and calorie deprivation may have led to a circumstance in which shivering is simply a waste of energy when sunrise will soon bring a source of warming exothermic energy. In the old traditions of Aborigines who sometimes take long treks through the arid "Outback" in central Australia, walking successfully from one area of the inland desert to another requires finding a source of water at least every 2–3 days to sustain life. In unfamiliar territory and lacking knowledge of where the next source of water might be, it is said that Aborigines use an exchange of information derived from their night-time dreams to arrive at a conclusion about the direction in which they should walk in order to find water. Rising from sleep somewhat hypothermic they gather around a fire in a circle to report to one another their recollections of dreams from the night. While everyone speaks and all dreams are relevant, it is thought that the dreams of the *children* are most important and weigh most heavily on group decision making. Children, it is said, have fresher imagination, less confusion about the reality of their dreams and are a more secure source of creative thoughts about the direction in which water may lie.

And so it may be with all of us who search and re-research, thirst and quest for new knowledge, committing our days to this quest as if new knowledge, like water, was essential to life itself. This we do in groups – sharing our dreams, exchanging our inspirations, listening intently to our young, and setting out daily in new directions on the journey we have chosen.

References

1. Oxford English Dictionary. Available at: www.oed.com/view/Entry/163433 (accessed June 28, 2012).
2. Blackburn RT, Lawrence JH. *Faculty at Work: motivation, expectation, satisfaction*. Baltimore, MD: Johns Hopkins University Press; 2002.

Index

Index

CASS (Coronary Artery Surgery Study) 153

CCM (chronic care model) 51, 58

CDC (Centers for Disease Control and Prevention) 50, 56, 61–2

cerebrospinal fluid 22

change
- management of 184
- stages of 60

CHARGE (Cohorts for Heart and Aging Research in Genomic Epidemiology)
- CHRU role in 147
- design of 160–1
- infrastructure grant 5, 143–4
- junior investigators in 161–2

check-ins 125, 136, 138

CHEP (Community Health Enhancement Program) 28–9

China
- economic reforms in 83, 87
- equipment sharing in 189–90
- PI system in 79–81
- research and development in 76–7, 80, 82–6, 98
- scientific journals in 83–4
- translational research in 17

Chinese Science and Technology Data Directory 83

Chlamydia screening 43, 53, 56

CHRU (Cardiovascular Health Research Unit)
- foundation of 146
- funding from 7, 144
- international collaboration of 159–60
- research culture of 164
- research projects of 148–50
- success of 147

CHS (Cardiovascular Health Study)
- and CHARGE 161
- Coordinating Center 154
- design of 147, 153
- "Future of" proposal 155–7
- publications by 157–8, **158**
- working groups of 154–5, 157, 161

Clinical Effectiveness Program, Harvard 6, 93

clinical research
- and competition for resources 42
- data analysis for 28, 106
- efficiency of 19, 37
- ethics of 32
- meaningful questions for 81

and networking 106–7
summer programs for 34, 97–105, **104**
teaching skills for 5, 8, 96–8, 107

CMMI (Center for Medicare and Medicaid Innovation) 59

cohort studies
- in cardiovascular disease 148, 160
- coordination across 162
- researcher–participant relationship in 64
- use of 103

collaboration
- cross-generational 146
- culture of 4

collaborative research
- and biostatistics 146
- culture of 153–4
- disincentives for 121
- in practice 43, 49, 53
- in project design 8
- and RCCRN 133–4

collaborators, critical characteristics of 3

Collins, Francis 43, 67

communication
- relationship-centered 123
- and science success 4

communities
- emergence of 190
- identifying needs in 95
- self-organizing 136

community-based participatory research 131

Community Health Enhancement Program (CHEP) 28–9, 32–3

community partnerships, and Indiana CTSI 28

complexity science 192

concept mapping 171

connectivity, value of 19

consent, informed 45, 145

Copass, Michael 144, 152

creativity
- and interpersonal relationships 137
- transformational 115

CRN (Cancer Research Network) 50, 61–2

crowdsourcing 18

CTSAs (Clinical and Translational Science Awards)
- and Group Health 66
- and Indiana 24–5, 27–8, 30
- funding of 19, 190

Index